Tinnitus Retraining Therapy

CLINICAL GUIDELINES

Editor-in-Chief for Audiology
Brad A. Stach, PhD

Tinnitus Retraining Therapy

CLINICAL GUIDELINES

James A. Henry, PhD
Dennis R. Trune, PhD, MBA
Michael J. A. Robb, MD
Pawel J. Jastreboff, PhD, ScD, MBA

Illustrations by Lynn H. Kitagawa, MFA

PLURAL PUBLISHING INC.
SAN DIEGO
OXFORD
BRISBANE

PLURAL PUBLISHING
INC.

5521 Ruffin Road
San Diego, CA 92123

e-mail: info@pluralpublishing.com
Web site: http://www.pluralpublishing.com

49 Bath Street
Abingdon, Oxfordshire OX14 1EA
United Kingdom

Typeset in 11/13 Garamond by Flanagan's Publishing Services, Inc.
Printed in the United States of America by McNaughton and Gunn

ISBN-13: 978-1-59756-154-9
ISBN-10: 1-59756-154-1

Library of Congress Cataloging-in-Publication Data

Tinnitus retraining therapy : clinical guidelines / James Henry . . . [et al.].
p. ; cm.
Includes bibliographical references and index.
ISBN-13: 978-1-59756-154-9 (softcover : alk. paper)
ISBN-10: 1-59756-154-1 (softcover : alk. paper)
1. Tinnitus. 2. Tinnitus–Treatment. I. Henry, James, 1949-
[DNLM: 1. Tinnitus–therapy. WV 272 T59177 2007]
RF293.8.T5667 2007
617.8–dc22

2006103494

Contents

Foreword

In 1975 I was introduced to the first effective treatment for tinnitus by Jack Vernon in Portland, Oregon. In 1987, after more than 15 years of tinnitus research in the UK, I was to find the best solution yet in a chance meeting with Pawel Jastreboff, and in my introduction to the neurophysiological model of tinnitus that he had already devised. My team in London began the first early implementation of the model in 1988, which with Pawel's help and guidance developed rapidly into Tinnitus Retraining Therapy (TRT) and resulted in 2004 in the publication of our seminal work on TRT by Cambridge University Press, UK. My continued friendship with Jack Vernon and his colleagues had renewed my contact with Jim Henry at the nearby Veterans Affairs Medical Center, who had been quick to use TRT to good advantage and produce the same excellent results that the pioneers had already experienced.

During discussions with Jim in the 1990s he was quick to identify the difficulties in teaching the model to patients, and also to professionals. The concepts of auditory neurophysiology were complex, were alien to audiology as it was taught at that time, and TRT needed to follow specific protocols to assure a highly successful treatment outcome.

Here Jim Henry is ably assisted by his co-authors, including the originator of the neuroscience behind TRT, Pawel Jastreboff, in a comprehensive 'How to do it' Tinnitus Retraining Therapy text book, which should not be purchased without the illustrated TRT counselling manual that goes with it.

The first of these books contains a review of the neurophysiological model with much scientific support and justification, as well as techniques and protocols for assessing and treating patients. It is an excellent introduction to the clinician and therapist making a start on TRT. This should always be viewed as a supplement to appropriate courses and in-service training, as in any area of audiological practice. Be prepared to find that TRT is effective and rewarding, but also demanding and challenging. Clinicians should avail themselves of all available resources to become skilled in the practice of TRT.

The second book is a wonderful compilation of diagrams and anatomical and physiological drawings to facilitate this teaching. It is comprehensive, covering almost every possible manifestation of tinnitus and hyperacusis that a professional and patient will meet. Careful selection of the teaching material is essential in dealing with individual cases. I am delighted to see the incorporation of some of the teaching material that both Pawel and I used ourselves for many years, but I wish I could have had this book at my side during my 18 years of TRT practice.

Jonathan W. P. Hazell, FRCS,
Director
Tinnitus and Hyperacusis Centre (ret.),
and Honary Consultant Surgeon,
University College London Hospitals,
London UK

Acknowledgments

The authors gratefully acknowledge the individuals who have contributed to the development of this book. All illustrations were developed by VA medical illustrator Lynn Kitagawa, MFA (Portland VA Medical Center—PVAMC) with full support from Medical Media Service at the PVAMC. Martin Schechter, PhD (PVAMC Audiology Clinic) and Tara Zaugg, AuD (VA National Center for Rehabilitative Auditory Research—NCRAR) have made innumerable contributions, especially with respect to assessment procedures and the questionnaire forms. Daniel Storzbach, PhD (PVAMC Mental Health Clinic) and Mitchel Turbin, PhD (NCRAR) contributed information about mental health referrals in Chapter 7 (Referral Guidelines). Laurence McKenna, PhD (Royal National Throat, Nose and Ear Hospital, London) and Christopher Cunningham, PhD (Chair, Behavioral Neuroscience, Oregon Health & Science University) critically reviewed Chapter 6 (Learning and Memory).

Stephen Fausti, PhD (Director, NCRAR) has provided ongoing advocacy and support of tinnitus research and educational activities at the NCRAR. Sara Ruth Oliver, AuD (Chief, PVAMC Audiology and Speech Pathology Service) has been a consistent supporter of NCRAR tinnitus research and education. Christine Kaelin, MBA (NCRAR) and Kimberly Owens, BS (NCRAR) have been "in the trenches" supporting every aspect of the NCRAR tinnitus research program.

We also thank the following individuals for their contributions: Terry D. Fife, MD, Konstantin Baev, PhD, Molly Harrington, MLS, AHIP, and Irma Contreras, assistant librarian (all at Barrow Neurological Institute/St. Joseph Hospital and Medical Center, Phoenix, Arizona) for helpful comments and assistance.

A special acknowledgment goes to Mary Jo Henry, who has personally supported this project in many ways.

Funding for this work was provided in part by Veterans Affairs Rehabilitation Research and Development (RR&D) Service (C3469S) (JAH), the RR&D National Center for Rehabilitative Auditory Research (C2659C) (JAH), and the NIH—National Institute on Deafness and Other Communication Disorders (R01 DC005593) (DRT).

About the Authors

James A. Henry, PhD

Dr. Henry is a Research Career Scientist at the National Center for Rehabilitative Auditory Research, located at the Veterans Affairs Medical Center in Portland, Oregon. He is also Associate Professor at the Department of Otolaryngology, Head and Neck Surgery at Oregon Health & and Science University (OHSU) in Portland. Dr. Henry earned a master's degree in Audiology at Portland State University and a doctorate in Behavioral Neuroscience at OHSU. His research career has been dedicated primarily to the development, evaluation, and documentation of methods for tinnitus clinical management. He has conducted numerous research studies, including controlled clinical trials to evaluate the efficacy of Tinnitus Retraining Therapy.

Dennis R. Trune, PhD, MBA

Dr. Trune earned his doctorate in Anatomy from the Louisiana State University Medical Center in New Orleans (1979) and conducted his doctoral research at the Kresge Hearing Research Laboratory of the South. Following a three-year postdoctoral research fellowship in the Otological Research Laboratories (Department of Otolaryngology) at Ohio State University, he joined the Oregon Health & Science University (OHSU) in Portland in 1983. He currently is Professor of Otolaryngology and a research scientist at the Oregon Hearing Research Center at OHSU. His research interests include the impact of inflammatory disorders on the inner ear and the molecular mechanisms in the cochlea that are controlled by steroid therapies for immune-mediated hearing loss. He also holds a joint appointment to the Portland Veterans Affairs Medical Center as a research scientist in the Department of Immunology and the National Center for Rehabilitative Auditory Research.

Michael J. A. Robb, MD

Dr. Robb is a neurologist, oto-neurologist, and medical neuro-otologist in Phoenix, Arizona specializing in diseases and disorders of the ear and the brain. His professional training includes a bachelor of arts degree from Washington University in St. Louis, Missouri; Doctor of Medicine from the University of Santo Tomas, Manila, Philippines; Diploma in Clinical Neurology, Institute of Neurology, National Hospital for Neurology & Neurosurgery, Queen Square, London, UK; Residency in Neurology, University of Wisconsin-Madison; and the Fife Fellowship in Medical Neuro-Otology from the Barrow Neurological Institute/St. Joseph's Hospital & Medical Center. He is currently a member of the Board of Directors and the Scientific Advisory Committee of the American Tinnitus Association in Portland, Oregon. Dr. Robb is dedicated to the private practice of medicine, student teaching, and clinical research in tinnitus, hyperacusis, hearing, and balance disorders.

Pawel J. Jastreboff, PhD, ScD, MBA

Dr. Jastreboff is a Professor and Director of the Emory Tinnitus and Hyperacusis Center. After 8 years at Yale University and 8 years at the University of Maryland, where he established the Tinnitus and Hyperacusis Center, Dr. Jastreboff moved to Emory University in January 1999 to continue his research on tinnitus and to create the Emory Tinnitus and Hyperacusis Center. In 1988, on the basis of research on the physiological mechanisms of tinnitus, Dr. Jastreboff proposed a neurophysiological model of tinnitus and Tinnitus Retraining Therapy (TRT). He has also created an animal model of tinnitus, and his present research is aimed at delineating the mechanisms of tinnitus and designing new methods of tinnitus and hyperacusis alleviation. Dr. Jastreboff received a Ph.D. in Neuroscience and Doctor of Sciences Degree (Neuroscience) from the Polish Academy of Science. He did his Postdoctoral training at the University of Tokyo, Japan. In 2005, he received an M.B.A. from Goizueta Business School at Emory University. He holds Visiting Professor appointments at Yale University School of Medicine and at University College London and Middlesex Hospital, London, England.

About the Illustrator

Lynn H. Kitagawa, MFA

Ms. Kitagawa received her Bachelor of Arts in Biology at Lewis and Clark College, Portland Oregon. She has also earned a BFA in Fine Art at the Pacific NW College of Art in Portland OR, and an MFA in Medical and Biological Illustration at the University of Michigan, Ann Arbor. Since 1986, she has been employed as a medical illustrator by Medical Media Service at the Portland Veterans Affairs Medical Center and has been a drawing instructor in the Continuing Education program at the Pacific NW College of Art.

Introduction

Tinnitus Retraining Therapy (TRT) was conceived and developed by Dr. Pawel J. Jastreboff and is a clinical implementation of his "neurophysiological model of tinnitus." The neurophysiological model conceptualizes tinnitus as a neural signal that can have varying effects on the central nervous system. The model was created in the 1980s and formally presented in 1990 (P. J. Jastreboff, 1990). J. Hazell and J. Sheldrake started using TRT as a clinical technique in London in 1988. In 1990, the method was first implemented in the United States by P. J. Jastreboff at the University of Maryland in Baltimore. P. J. Jastreboff presently conducts research and directs a tinnitus treatment center at Emory University in Atlanta. Thousands of patients have received treatment at these clinics in London, Baltimore, and Atlanta. TRT is currently performed in well over 100 clinics around the world.

After its inception, interest in TRT grew rapidly, resulting in the need to train professionals in the methodology. In response to this need, J. Hazell began offering annual TRT training seminars in 1992. P. J. Jastreboff has conducted semiannual instructional courses since 1996. In addition, these founders of TRT have conducted numerous workshops in many countries.

Many articles about TRT have been written over the years (see, for example Hazell, 1998, 2002; P. J. Jastreboff, 1990, 2004; P. J. Jastreboff, Gray, & Gold, 1996; P. J. Jastreboff & Hazell, 1993; P. J. Jastreboff & M.M. Jastreboff, 2000, 2001). The reader is encouraged to refer to these and other articles written by P. J. Jastreboff and J. Hazell to obtain the most comprehensive understanding of TRT. A detailed description of TRT also is available in a recently published book (P. J. Jastreboff & Hazell, 2004).

In the United States, audiologists specialize in clinical services relating to the prevention, assessment, and rehabilitation of auditory and associated communication disorders. (Every country has health care professionals who serve in this role, although not all are called audiologists.) Audiologists have received the education and training, and have performed the types of clinical services, that position them as appropriate TRT practitioners (J. A. Henry, P. J. Jastreboff, M. M. Jastreboff, Schechter, & Fausti, 2002). Audiologists may in fact be the most qualified health care professionals to perform TRT due to the specific clinical services that are provided with TRT: (a) an audiological evaluation is required; (b) the counseling protocol involves a description of the auditory system and an explanation of patients' audiological test results; (c) many patients have hearing loss that must be treated in conjunction with TRT; and (d) ear-level devices, which often include amplification, are provided to patients who undergo long-term treatment with TRT. Non-audiologists can perform certain components of TRT, but the services of an audiologist would be required to fulfill all aspects of the program.

Part 1 of this book describes neural and learning principles that are consistent with the concepts conveyed during TRT counseling. Parts 2 and 3 provide detailed clinical guidelines for performing the different components of assessment and treatment, respectively, using TRT methodology. A suggested TRT counseling script is provided in Part 3, which corresponds directly with the patient counseling book (*Tinnitus Retraining Therapy: Patient Counseling Guide*) that was developed as a companion volume to this book. All of the information in both books would be considered complementary to the information that is contained in P. J. Jastreboff and J. Hazell's (2004) seminal book about TRT.

The method of TRT uses a structured protocol of educational counseling and sound therapy that requires a minimum of one year of treatment for patients with a severe condition. (Patients with less severe tinnitus require proportionally less treatment.) The counseling protocol is designed to remove any negative associations that patients may have with their tinnitus, including fears related to tinnitus. Successful treatment with TRT depends critically upon the clinician's competence in administering the counseling. TRT counseling amounts to an educational session—the clinician is the teacher and the patient is the student. The main elements of counseling are covered during the initial treatment visit and counseling is continuous at return visits. The effectiveness of TRT depends on the effectiveness of the counseling. It is thus essential that the clinician possesses a thorough understanding of the principles of TRT, as well as the ability to convey this information effectively to patients in a compassionate, authoritative, and unhurried manner. Most importantly, patients must clearly understand the neurophysiological model of tinnitus (P. J. Jastreboff, 1990; P. J. Jastreboff & Hazell, 2004), which is the essence of TRT. Effective teaching of the model and the other unique concepts of TRT requires the clinician to acquire a conversant understanding about certain nonauditory brain systems, in addition to relevant principles of learning.

TRT counseling always includes an explanation of "sound therapy" and the rationale for its use. All patients treated with TRT must be informed of the need to enrich their sound environments with the proper type of sound to facilitate the treatment goals. For patients requiring long-term treatment, sound therapy usually includes the use of ear-level devices (sound generators, hearing aids, or combination instruments containing both noise generation and amplification).

The clinical goals of TRT are twofold: habituation of reactions to tinnitus and habituation of the tinnitus perception. These two interrelated objectives are accomplished through the neural mechanism of habituation, which is a natural learning process whereby repeated exposure to an innocuous stimulus results in a decreased response to the stimulus. The stimulus in this case is tinnitus, and the ultimate aim of TRT is for patients to habituate the tinnitus. To achieve habituation, the tinnitus neural signal must be "reclassified" to the status of a meaningless auditory signal, such as the continuous sound from an air conditioning vent, computer/electric fan, or a refrigerator.

The first and most important goal of TRT is habituation of *reactions* to tinnitus. These reactions involve predominantly the sympathetic part of the autonomic nervous system (which mediates stress-related responses) that is controlled by the limbic system (which mediates emotions). Habituation of the *perception* of tinnitus is the secondary goal, and will follow automatically once habituation of reactions is achieved to a sufficient degree. When both goals are achieved, patients are aware of their tinnitus for a very small percentage of their waking hours, and when they are aware of it, the tinnitus is not (or is only mildly) bothersome. Thus, when they attend to their tinnitus, emotional and autonomic reactions are eliminated, or at least minimized.

It is well accepted that approximately 80% of individuals who experience chronic tinnitus do not require clinical intervention (A. Davis & Refaie, 2000; P. J. Jastreboff & Hazell, 2004). For the remaining 20%, some degree of clinical intervention is necessary, ranging from a single counseling session to long-term therapy (Dobie, 2004b). Long-term treatment with TRT is warranted only for patients who think about their tinnitus and react to it to such a degree that their quality of life is significantly reduced. Individuals who are the most bothered by their tinnitus may be the ones who receive the greatest benefit from TRT (J. A. Henry et al., 2006a,b).

The purpose of this book, and its companion volume, is to provide clinical tools to TRT professionals to assist them in administering TRT to their patients as consistently and effectively as possible. The effectiveness of TRT requires a thorough clinical assessment, adherence to the treatment protocol, and knowledge of the neurological bases for tinnitus and for the neurophysiological model. The most essential element of TRT is the counseling protocol (P. J. Jastreboff, 1995), which is most effective when the clinician has a solid grasp of the underlying neurological principles of the model. It is our assertion that TRT professionals who understand these principles and employ the prescribed clinical protocol will maximize their effectiveness in rendering treatment to patients whose lives have been significantly impacted by tinnitus.

This book is dedicated to tinnitus patients everywhere,
and to the clinicians and researchers who are dedicated to helping them.

PART 1

Neural and Learning Principles of TRT

Effective patient counseling for TRT requires the practitioner to understand the neurophysiological bases for tinnitus, its perception, tinnitus-induced reactions, and potential mechanisms for its control. Part 1 provides a foundation for TRT that supplements the background information provided by P. J. Jastreboff and Hazell (2004). In Part 1, theories consistent with the neurophysiological model of TRT are described and illustrated for brain centers involved in tinnitus perception and control. Part 1 concludes with a chapter that explains learning and conditioning principles and their theoretical application to tinnitus as a neural "stimulus," as well as how TRT clinicians utilize these principles during treatment. The presentation of these concepts should be tailored in unique ways to yield optimum patient understanding and response to treatment.

1

Neuroanatomy and Neurophysiology

Tinnitus is a neural signal in the brain that the patient consciously perceives as sound. The signal can also cause emotional reactions. Effective treatment with TRT requires a reduction in both these behaviors. The brain is a very sophisticated sensory integration organ that allows us to not only consciously perceive our environment, but also subconsciously adapt to sensations that are irrelevant or unnecessary. Thus, the brain devotes "attention" to those important sensations requiring a reaction while simultaneously ignoring environmental information that is not important. One of the main detrimental actions of tinnitus is that it dominates attention, which interferes with other important behavioral activities or emotions. The objective of intervention is to cause the brain to switch its focus away from the tinnitus neural signal and process it like an irrelevant auditory signal. This is the basis for TRT. TRT is effective because it exploits these natural neural networks of the brain that are responsible for processing sensory information by forcing them to relegate any response to tinnitus to the subconscious. Thus, tinnitus does not go away, but the brain stops reacting to it and ceases attending to it.

NERVE CELLS

Every part of the body is composed of cells. Brain cells are called neurons (or nerve cells) and are different from other cells primarily because they communicate directly with each other (LeDoux, 2002). The point of communication is called the synapse, which is a highly developed system of membrane specializations that allows neurochemical transmitters to move between the connected nerve cells. The human brain contains over 100 billion individual neurons and most of these have thousands of synapses.

The cell body of most neurons has numerous branches (dendrites) that receive incoming signals from other nerve cells (Figure 1-1). The neuron also has an axon that transmits nerve impulses away from the cell body to synapse with other neurons. Axons typically have a whitish appearance due to their insulative coating of fatty myelin to increase conduction speed (not all axons are covered by myelin). Hence, areas of the brain occupied by axon tracts appear white (white matter), while areas occupied predominantly by neuron cell bodies are gray (gray matter).

Every nerve cell has only one axon, but this axon often branches to end in multiple terminals on multiple neurons (LeDoux, 2002). This branching architecture of the axon allows a message (impulse) from one neuron to form synapses with as many as 1,000 other neurons, generally on their dendrites (Kandel, 2000d). Because of the branching dendrites, each neuron can receive signals from thousands of other neurons—some receive over 100,000 synaptic inputs (Vander, Sherman, & Luciano, 1990). There are on average tens of thousands of connections for every neuron (Amaral, 2000). The number of connections

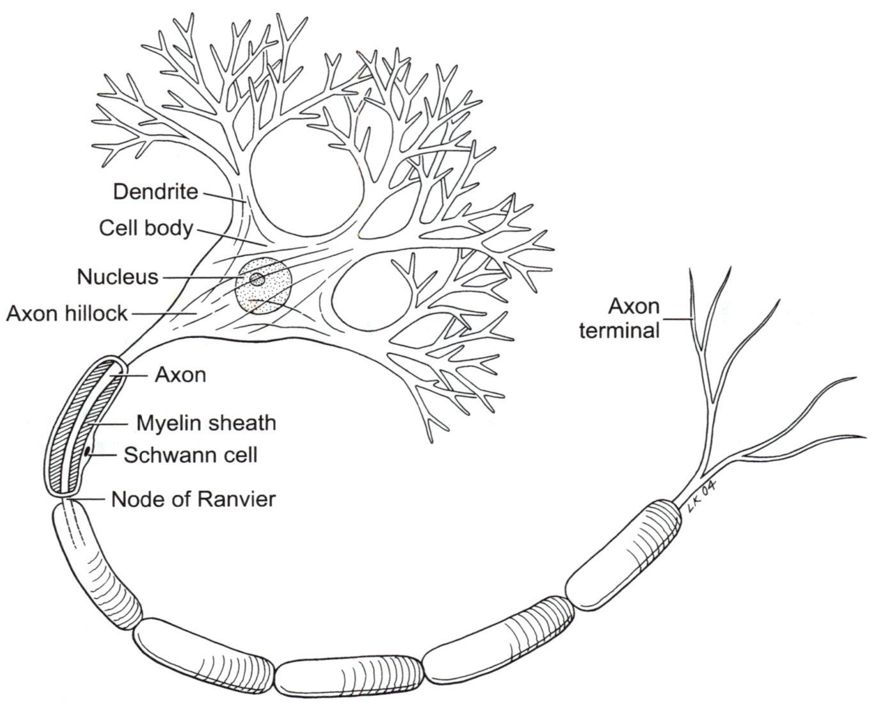

FIGURE 1–1. Basic structure of neurons.

(synapses) in the human brain is incomprehensively large. If every connection could be listed in a series of books, it would require 500 libraries the size of the largest library in the world (the Library of Congress in Washington, D.C., that contains about 20 million volumes) to contain the full set of books describing all of the direct connections in a single human brain (Gitt, 1999).

Although there are at least 1,000 different types of neurons, they all share the same basic mechanism of electrical signaling (Kandel, 2000d). Information transmission and processing by neurons is mediated by electrical signals called action potentials, which are all-or-none nerve impulses that are triggered at the initial segment of the axon (axon hillock) (Figure 1-1). The impulse is conducted down the axon at speeds of 1 to 100 meters per second (corresponding to 2 to 224 miles per hour) and with a constant amplitude of about 100 mV. Neurons are very active metabolically compared to most tissue—the human nervous system comprises only 1 to 2% of the body's weight, yet it consumes close to 25% of the body's caloric energy (Anderson, 1995).

Neurons have threshold levels of excitation that determine whether or not they will fire an action potential. In the resting state, neurons are polarized with respect to their immediate environment, i.e., the inside of the cell membrane is negatively charged relative to the outside. Ion "pumps" are protein channels distributed throughout the membrane that pump ions through the membrane in the direction necessary to maintain this resting polarization. Cells must be depolarized (i.e., potential has to increase) to their threshold level to trigger a sudden influx of sodium (Na^+) ions through Na^+ channels, which generates an action potential (Kandel, 2000d). The initial uninsulated portion of an axon (axon hillock) has the lowest threshold because it contains the highest density of these voltage-sensitive Na^+ channels. In this "trigger zone" of the axon, all of the input signals are summed, and excitation occurs if the sum of the signals reaches the depolarization threshold. The excitation is all-or-none. The only information an element can communicate to other connected elements is represented in this all-or-none event (Carlson, 1991).

NEURAL NETWORKS

All nerve cells have similar basic properties, but they produce different actions according to their particular connections (Kandel, 2000d; LeDoux, 2002). The key to how neurons coordinate the brain's efficient system of communication lies in the patterns of connections between nerve cells, which form precise anatomical circuits that function using parallel processing (Figure 1-2). The brain consists of networks of neurons, and information processing and learning occur in these "neural networks" (Carlson, 1991). Single cells are not capable of initiating complex human behaviors; these can only be generated by the coordinated actions of many cells (Kandel, 2000d). Computer modeling of neural networks simulates the summing action of signals that are responsible for generating action potentials—a response occurs only if the sum of the weighted inputs exceeds the activation threshold. This same process occurs with each element that is contained within the network.

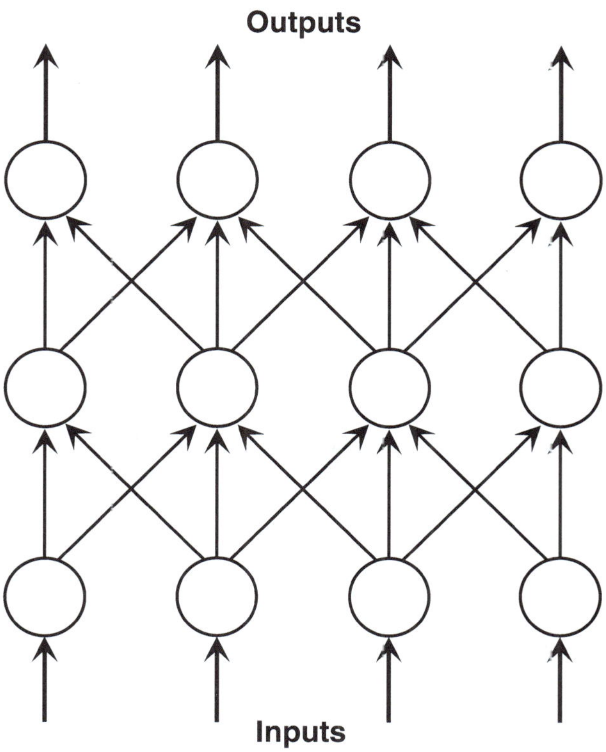

FIGURE 1–2. Network of interconnected units, depicting how the brain performs parallel processing of neural information.

Neural networks acquire the ability to recognize specific stimuli (Carlson, 1991). When an unfamiliar stimulus pattern is presented to a network, the outputs from the network will be weak and nonspecific. If the same pattern is presented repeatedly, a specific output pattern will be produced that is strong and reliable. In this manner, unique output patterns are developed for each stimulus pattern that is presented repeatedly to the network. Neural networks are then capable of discriminating between incoming stimulus patterns that are recognizable (Anderson, 1995). Networks also have the ability to generalize, i.e., to respond appropriately to stimulus patterns that are novel but similar to recognizable patterns. This ability to generalize is one of the great strengths of neural networks.

The counseling protocol for TRT incorporates a brief description of neural networks. This helps the patient understand how the brain normally processes sensory signals, and how neural networks also process the neural tinnitus signal (tinnitus-related neural activity) *as if* it was a representation of an auditory signal reaching the inner ear. Thus, the brain cannot distinguish between a "phantom" auditory signal that is internally generated and a signal that has been coded to represent some sound generated outside the inner ear. Whether internally or externally generated, the final common pathway for tinnitus perception is the neural network that processes auditory signals to the level of consciousness. Therefore, the counselor must understand the central nervous system regions that contain the neural networks responsible for processing tinnitus signals.

THE BRAIN

The central nervous system (CNS) is composed of the spinal cord and the brain (Figure 1-3). The brain can be divided into six main parts called medulla, pons, midbrain, cerebellum, diencephalon, and cerebral hemispheres (Amaral, 2000; Kandel, 2000a). Although these brain regions are

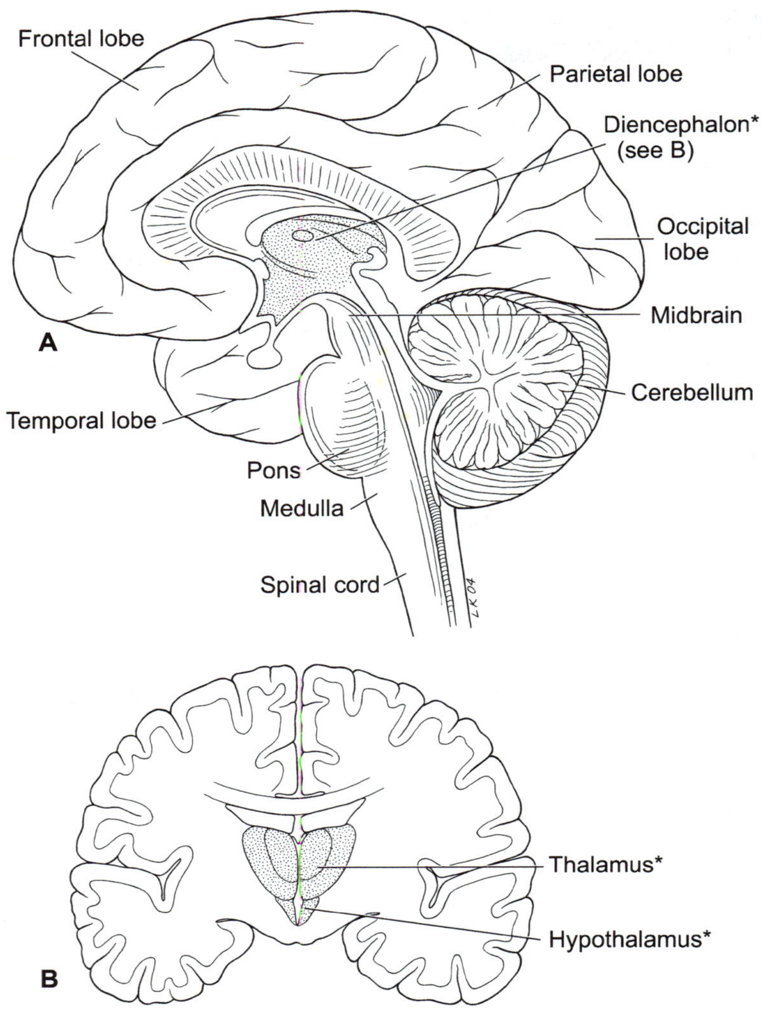

FIGURE 1–3. Major structures of the brain. **A.** Midsagittal view. **B.** Coronal section at level of diencephalon.

given different names, the CNS is a series of ascending (sensory) pathways and descending (motor) pathways that run between the spinal cord and cerebral cortex. Information processed by these pathways is often modified by other neural centers or networks as it passes through these brain regions. An overview of these different brain parts is provided below, with greater emphasis on structures that are most relevant to TRT.

The central auditory pathway is comprised of multiple nuclei and nerve tracts that run the entire length of the brain to terminate in the auditory cortex. All auditory nerve fibers synapse on neurons within the cochlear nucleus, but from here secondary neurons project to multiple areas of the brainstem, such as the superior olivary complex, nuclei of the lateral lemniscus, and the inferior colliculus (Figure 1-4). Third order neurons in the superior olivary complex and nuclei of the lateral lemniscus then project to the inferior colliculus. Neurons within the inferior colliculus send axons to the medial geniculate body in the thalamus, which in turn projects to the primary auditory cortex. Although these nuclear centers process sound information for conscious awareness, auditory pathway fibers also project into areas of the brain not traditionally thought of as related to hearing, such as the reticular formation, superior colliculus, cerebellum, amygdala, etc. (Please refer to Figures 1-3 and 1-4 throughout this chapter.)

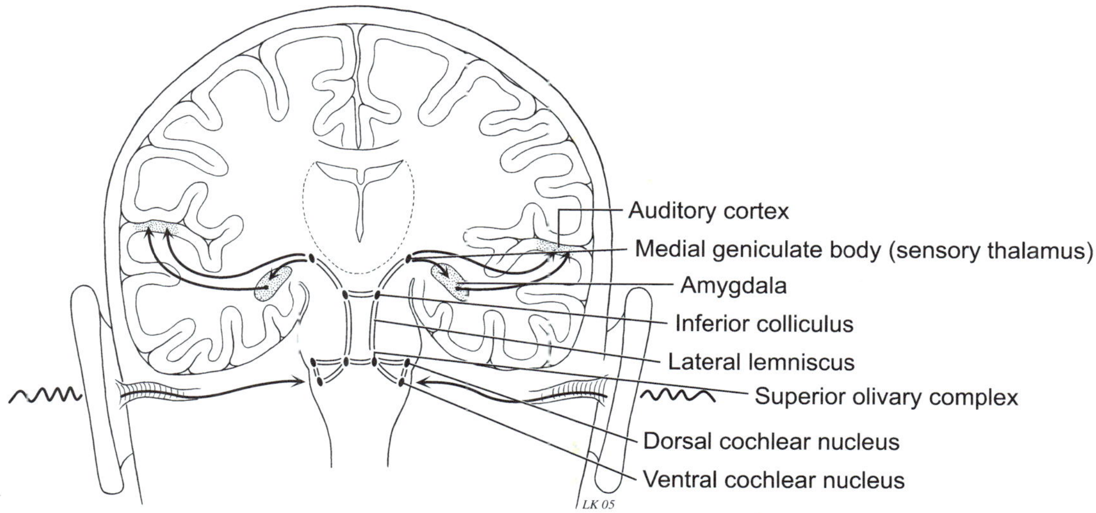

FIGURE 1–4. Central auditory pathways.

Medulla

The medulla, pons, and midbrain comprise the brainstem. The brainstem integrates inputs and outputs from cranial nerves II–XII and is responsible for critical sensory and motor functions. The medulla is the transition from the spinal cord to the brain and contains nuclear centers that control life-support functions such as blood pressure, heart rate, breathing, and digestion. There also are neuronal groups in the medulla that serve as initial relay stations for most sensations, including hearing. The auditory nerve enters the brainstem (just below the juncture between the medulla and the pons) to synapse in the cochlear nucleus. Thus, the first processing within the "auditory network" occurs here.

Pons

Moving up the brainstem, the medulla transitions into the pons. The pons contains cell groups that convey information about voluntary motor movement from the cerebral cortex to the cerebellum (Amaral, 2000; Kandel, 2000a). Other cell groups in the pons are involved in sensory and motor functions of the face, eye movements, hearing and balance, control of breathing, taste, and sleep. The superior olivary complex is the first auditory center whose neurons receive input from both ears and is part of the neural network for localizing sound.

Midbrain

The third brainstem structure is the midbrain, located between the pons and the diencephalon. The midbrain contains cell groups that are responsible for controlling many sensory and motor functions, including the coordination of auditory reflexes (Amaral, 2000). The inferior colliculus is located in the midbrain and is another center for integration of input from the two ears.

Cerebellum

The cerebellum—the "mini-brain" at the back of the brainstem (posterior cranial fossa)—works in conjunction with the pons, basal ganglia, premotor cortex, and motor cortex to control skeletal (voluntary) muscles. Skilled actions, such as performing a sport or playing a musical instrument, require rapid movements that are smooth and accurate. The cerebellum coordinates these fine muscular movements and the learning of motor skills (Amaral, 2000; Kandel, 2000a). The cerebellum has strong auditory input (P. J. Jastreboff &

Tarnecki, 1975; Mathiak, Hertrich, Grodd, & Ackermann, 2002; Woody, Wang, & Gruen, 1998), the role of which still is not clear (P. J. Jastreboff, 1981; Oertel & Young, 2004). The cerebellum also has recently been discovered to be involved in language and other cognitive functions. The main control of cognitive function, however, occurs in the cerebral hemispheres, which form the largest of the six parts of the brain.

Diencephalon

The diencephalon includes the thalamus and the hypothalamus. Each of these structures is critically important to the concepts of TRT.

Thalamus

Sensory information (other than olfactory) travels through the thalamus on its way to perception regions in the cerebral hemispheres (Amaral, 2000; Kandel, 2000a). The thalamus gates and modulates this information by determining whether or not the input signals will reach cortical areas of conscious awareness. The medial geniculate body is the main relay center of auditory input to the primary auditory cortex in the temporal lobe. Specific regions of the thalamus also are responsible for gating auditory signals, including tinnitus. For example, the thalamus, and especially the medial geniculate body, conveys auditory signals to the amygdala (one of the main structures of the limbic system) (Cacace, 2004; LeDoux, Farb, Ruggiero, & Reis, 1987; Møller, 2003). P. J. Jastreboff (2000, p. 366) noted:

> The neuronal networks composing the central nervous system have the ability to selectively enhance or suppress a specific pattern of neuronal activity (Pribram, 1987). Consequently, it is possible for such a network to selectively block, filter-out, tinnitus related activity while not changing the processing of other patterns of activity. Specifically, the networks providing the limbic system with auditory information (connections between the medial geniculate body and the amygdala) are involved.

Thus, these centers play a vital role in habituation of the tinnitus, which will be discussed in detail later.

Hypothalamus

The peanut-sized hypothalamus has extensive connections with most areas of the CNS and is the key brain structure for regulating autonomic, endocrine, and visceral function (Amaral, 2000; Kandel, 2000a). The hypothalamus provides overall control of the autonomic nervous system and is responsible for maintaining homeostasis (stable internal body conditions). Secretion of hormones by the pituitary gland is regulated directly by the hypothalamus, which exerts control over growth, eating, drinking, and maternal behavior. The hypothalamus also is critically involved in initiating and controlling behaviors that are considered rewarding, such as hunger and sex. Notably, it also controls responses to threat.

Cerebral Hemispheres

The cerebral hemispheres contain the cerebral cortex with its underlying white matter (axon tracts), as well as the deep-lying basal nuclei, amygdala, and hippocampal formation (Amaral, 2000; Kandel, 2000a). (Note: Technically, *basal nuclei* is the correct terminology, not *basal ganglia*, since this structure is contained in the CNS. Ganglia are peripheral nervous system structures. The term *basal ganglia* has stuck erroneously through the years in texts and lectures.) In addition to cognitive functions of memory and emotion, the cerebral hemispheres are responsible for conscious sensation, voluntary motor control, language, behavior, and special talents in music and mathematics. The basal nuclei contribute to the control of fine movement. The amygdala is the key structure involved with learning and expression of emotion. The hippocampus is associated mostly with memory function. Commissures are neural links between similar regions of the two sides of the brain. The corpus callosum, containing 100 million fibers, is by far the largest of the commissures.

Cerebral Cortex

The cerebral cortex makes up the surface layer of the cerebral hemispheres. It is a sheet of deeply fissured and convoluted gray matter (neurons) that encompasses the region of conscious activity. The folds and convolutions triple the surface area of the cortex (only one-third of the cortex is exposed on the surface), allowing it to be packed densely into the restricted volume of the skull (Brodal, 2004). Although only an eighth of an inch thick, the cortex makes up more than half of all gray matter in the CNS and contains about 20 billion neurons—thus indicating its functional importance. The temporal lobe contains primary auditory cortex, which is responsible for awareness of sound. The temporal lobe also contains centers for memory. Association tracts interconnect many of these different cortical regions to integrate memory with sensations of hearing, vision, taste, etc. This integrative network plays a key role in TRT, particularly efforts to control the conscious perception of tinnitus and responses to it.

2

Consciousness

Consciousness can be defined simplistically as a "state of awareness" (Kandel, 2000c). The secondary goal of treatment with TRT is to remove the tinnitus signal from this state of awareness. Most processing of information in the brain occurs at a nonconscious level, and only some end products of these processes reach consciousness (Kihlstrom, 1987; LeDoux, 2000). There are numerous factors that determine whether or not sensory information (including the sensation of tinnitus) enters consciousness. We will discuss several of those factors below, such as working memory and directed attention.

With chronic tinnitus, the tinnitus-related neural signal is continually active at subconscious levels. It is important to understand that the signal does not have to enter consciousness to cause negative reactions. Learning (including the creation of conditioned reflexes) can occur at conscious and/or subconscious levels. Learning of emotional reactions is primarily a subconscious process. The sensory thalamus and the amygdala are directly connected (Cacace, 2004; LeDoux, 1992, 1998; LeDoux et al., 1987; Møller, 2003), which is the primary circuit for the subconscious learning of emotional reactions. Thus, when tinnitus causes emotional reactions, the reactions are mediated by subconscious circuits (loops) that have been established by the association of tinnitus with negative experiences. Activation of these loops, as governed by conditioned reflex principles, is in itself sufficient for tinnitus-induced distress (P. J. Jastreboff & Hazell, 2004). As such, the principal goal of TRT is habituation of these reactions, which requires "retraining" of the underlying circuits. All of these concepts will be discussed later in Part 1. First, however, we will discuss consciousness and directed attention, and how these cognitive processes relate to tinnitus perception.

WORKING MEMORY

The "state of awareness" definition of consciousness begs the question, "Aware of what?" LeDoux (1998) states that consciousness is "awareness of what is in working memory." The concept of working memory is the basis for many recent theories about consciousness. LeDoux describes working memory as a "mental workspace" that involves the temporary storage and active processing of memories and sensory information to facilitate thinking and reasoning. This processing is mediated by a network of interconnected brain regions that are described below. Working memory should be distinguished from short-term memory, which refers to a more restricted system of temporary information storage. Working memory implies an active processing mechanism that interrelates various pieces of information to facilitate cognition.

Components of Working Memory

There are numerous theories about working memory, but they all assume the existence of some kind of master controller that directs and coordinates conscious activity (LeDoux, 1998). This concept of a master controller is perhaps the most abstract and intangible aspect of consciousness that eludes any rational explanation. Its manifestation is recognized as focused, or directed, attention. We will have much more to say about directed attention in the next chapter, but for now we will assume that there is some mechanism that controls all of the mental activities necessary to focus attention on a given task. The operations involved in computer function offer numerous analogies to the various components of working memory. Whatever takes place in a computer is wholly directed by which keys are depressed on the keyboard. The master controller of working memory is whatever is behind the selection of the different "mental keystrokes."

The master controller requires an area in which to work, and it is this workspace that is the core of working memory (LeDoux, 1998). Working memory is thus the hub of conscious activity. It is, in effect, a general-purpose temporary storage system where all of the various bits of mental information are collected, sorted, integrated, and outputted. In computer terminology, any temporary storage circuit is a "buffer." The general-purpose temporary storage mechanism that serves as the workspace for working memory is the main buffer, analogous to a computer's random access memory.

Working memory (the general-purpose buffer) must have information with which to work. This information comes from two sources: sensory information and long-term memory (LeDoux, 1998). The information from these two sources is made available to working memory as multiple specialized buffers (Figure 2–1). Each specialized buffer can contain a different kind of information (auditory, visual, semantic, numeric, etc.). It is thought that working memory has simultaneous access to a maximum of approximately seven pieces of information (or seven specialized buffers) (LeDoux, 1998; Miller, 1956). During conscious thought, each of these seven or so pieces of information is available to working memory, but only one can be most effectively accessed at a given moment (LeDoux, 1998). In considering what a *piece of information* means, it is important to realize that the amount of information contained in a specialized buffer can be enormous due to the availability of any long-term memories that are linked to the particular concept. This access to long-term memories enables conscious experience to be connected with past experiences, which is crucial for proper interpretation of events and appropriate decision-making. Consciousness is therefore dependent on the availability of long-term memories.

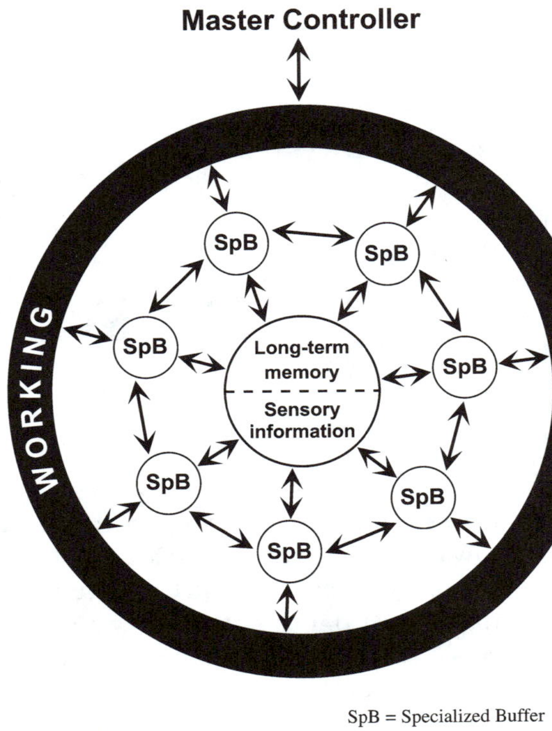

FIGURE 2–1. Working memory and its components. A master controller directs all activities of working memory. The working memory "workspace" has access to as many as seven (or more) specialized buffers that contain information drawn from sensory systems and from long-term memory (LeDoux, 1998; Miller, 1956).

Consciousness also requires active short-term memory processing. As an example, the auditory system has various temporary-storage buffers that assist in auditory perception by momentarily retaining different aspects of auditory information. The brain interprets auditory information by constantly comparing current with preceding auditory signals. When listening to a story, for example, its meaning can be understood only by remembering the first part of the story during the last part of the story.

Consciousness is a stream of mental processing that requires manipulation of a dynamic mechanism. As "one thought leads to another," active buffers are deactivated and replaced with newly activated buffers (LeDoux, 1998). Thus, the conscious mind is limited, but only in (a) the number of conscious experiences that can take place at a given instant (with one experience being dominant) and (b) the number of memories that are available to be drawn into consciousness.

Cortical Areas Involved in Working Memory

Although the neural substrate of the conscious state is unknown, it is known that the cerebral cortex is essential for the existence of consciousness (Brodal, 2004). The cerebral cortex is not, however, the only site of consciousness. Consciousness is "produced" through the interaction of the cortex and other parts of the brain. A critical interaction in this respect is the communication between the cortex and the thalamus.

Three areas of the frontal cortex have been implicated in the control of working memory: lateral prefrontal cortex, anterior cingulate cortex, and orbital region of the prefrontal cortex (Figure 2–2) (LeDoux, 1998). The lateral prefrontal cortex is most often implicated, with substantial evidence indicating its overall control of general-purpose working memory. Damage to this area results in impaired working-memory function regardless of the type of information being processed (Petrides, 1994). Anatomical connections of the lateral prefrontal cortex support its role as master controller of working memory—there are connections with the different sensory systems (including auditory), with areas involved in long-term memory, including the hippocampus, and with areas involved in short-term memory (Uylings & van Eden, 1990). Furthermore, the lateral prefrontal cortex has connections with cortical areas that control movement, enabling conscious thought to be turned into voluntary action (Fuster, 1989).

There also is evidence for involvement of the anterior cingulate cortex in control of working memory (Fuster, 1989; LeDoux, 1998). The anterior cingulate cortex and the lateral prefrontal cortex are anatomically interconnected, and they have been referred to as the "frontal lobe

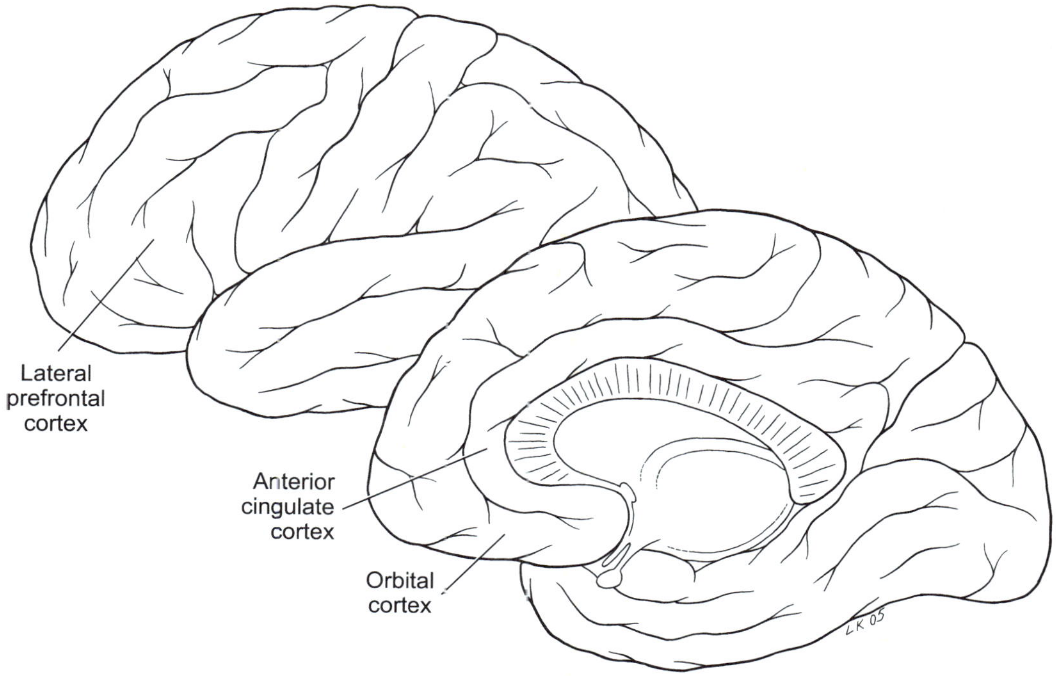

FIGURE 2–2. Cortical areas implicated in the control of working memory.

attentional network" (Posner & Driver, 1992). This network is thought to be involved in selective attention, decision-making, and control of voluntary movements. In addition, these two regions work together to coordinate the allocation of mental resources, i.e., to control which aspects of memory are involved at any given moment in conscious activity.

The third area of the frontal cortex that is involved in working memory is the orbital cortex (LeDoux, 1998). This area has connections with the anterior cingulate cortex, and also receives inputs from sensory systems. In addition, the amygdala projects to the orbital cortex (as well as to the anterior cingulate cortex), thus providing a link between emotional processing in the amygdala and conscious processing of sensory information. Damage to this area in humans causes a disruption in the ability to comprehend social and emotional cues, and can lead to sociopathic behavior and seizures.

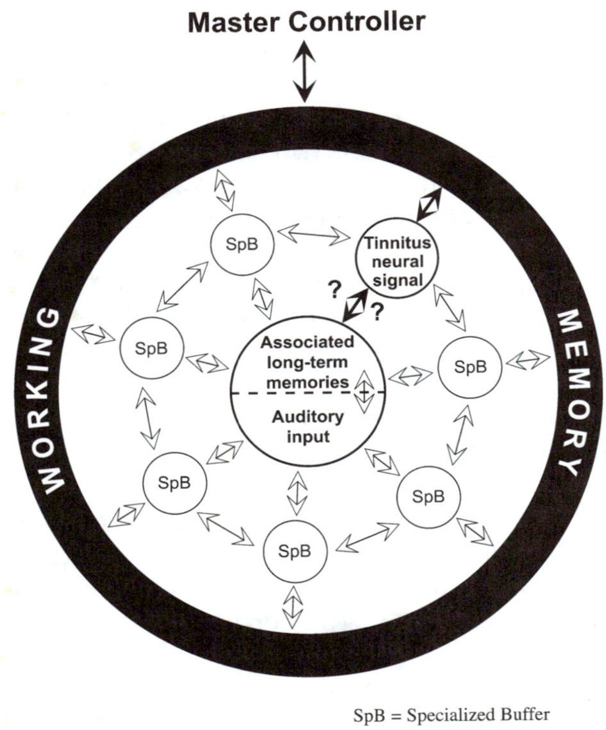

FIGURE 2–3. Conceptual relationship between the tinnitus-related neural signal and working memory. The tinnitus neural signal is shown as occupying one of the specialized memory buffers that is being accessed preferentially by working memory. Long-term memories may or may not be associated with the tinnitus, as indicated by the question marks. Also, there is the potential for the tinnitus signal to be affected by sensory input, especially auditory input.

Working Memory and Tinnitus

As explained above, all of the activity that takes place within the hub of working memory is coordinated by a master controller (see Figure 2-1) (LeDoux, 1998). The controller determines which specialized memory buffers are active at a given moment and how the buffers interact with each other. With respect to tinnitus, the tinnitus neural signal would occupy a single, independent memory buffer (Figure 2-3). Conscious attention being given to tinnitus would mean that the master controller has directed the tinnitus buffer into the working-memory workspace. If the tinnitus buffer has no associated memories, then the conscious tinnitus perception would simply comprise one of as many as seven pieces of information immediately accessible to the conscious mind. A tinnitus signal with no associated memories would be perceived as a formless auditory pattern that is devoid of meaning.

On the other hand, if long-term memories are associated with the tinnitus, activation of the tinnitus buffer might secondarily activate those memories (Figure 2-3). Activation of any associated unpleasant memories could cause negative emotional and autonomic reactions. In Chapter 4 we will discuss neural mechanisms of emotions and how they interrelate with the perception of the tinnitus signal. In essence, if the associated emotional memories are particularly strong, conscious activity could become dominated by the memories. In such a case, the tinnitus neural signal has gained the full attention of the master controller, which retains the tinnitus in working memory—potentially resulting in a chronic emotional state that is dominated by the tinnitus perception.

The tinnitus buffer also can be influenced by sensory input, especially from the auditory system (Figure 2-3). Auditory input can have various effects on the perception of tinnitus. First, the input could make the tinnitus signal inaudible. Such an effect has been termed *tinnitus masking*, but at the neural level it is more appropriately termed *suppression* of tinnitus (P. J. Jastreboff & Hazell, 2004; P. J. Jastreboff & M. M. Jastreboff, 2001). Alternatively, the auditory input may be perceptible but not decrease the tinnitus perception. When this occurs, the net result is that the signal-to-noise (tinnitus to background sound) ratio has been reduced. This points to a critical concept regarding the use of sound therapy with TRT—background sound should be maintained, but without changing the tinnitus perception (timbre). When raised to a certain level, the auditory input will start to alter the tinnitus perception, at which point the two signals start to blend or mix together. The discussion of habituation in Chapter 6 will include an explanation of the theory that the tinnitus perception must be unchanged for habituation to be most effective. In effect, if the tinnitus signal is changed perceptually the tendency will be for habituation to occur to this modified tinnitus signal. Then, when the "usual" tinnitus perception returns after removal of the additional sound, habituation to this usual/baseline tinnitus will be only partial due to the generalization principle. Thus, sound levels above the "mixing point" still produce some habituation due to generalization, but this is not the optimal approach (P. J. Jastreboff, 2000; P. J. Jastreboff & Hazell, 2004). The mixing point is the threshold level at which external sound just begins to cause a perceived spectral change in the tinnitus (a change in timbre). With TRT, the use of external sound must be at or below the mixing point for optimal effectiveness. (See Chapter 13 for a full explanation of the mixing point and related concepts.)

3

Directed Attention

Directed attention refers to the ability to focus on stimuli that are important while avoiding distraction by irrelevant stimuli (Vander et al., 1990). This ability requires the nervous system to continuously evaluate the importance of incoming sensory information.

NEURAL MECHANISMS OF DIRECTED ATTENTION

One of the unique attributes of consciousness is its unity of function (Kandel, 2000c). That is, conscious perception amounts to a singular experience derived from the coordinated integration of all the events occurring at a given instant in the CNS. All of this neural activity must be routed in such a way as to facilitate focused attention on the present activity. Millions of sensory receptors flood the brain constantly with impulses, most of which must be suppressed at a subconscious level because they are not immediately relevant. Only a small fraction of the stimuli are relevant to a given situation and must be appropriately routed to provide the consciousness with the information necessary to execute its unique role. The brain must therefore perform a filtering function to differentiate important from unimportant stimuli. This filtering has to be performed at a subconscious level and is accomplished mainly by the reticular formation, which will be described following a description of general mechanisms of attention.

General Mechanisms of Selective Attention

All sensory systems have a common signaling mechanism that involves sensory receptors as the first in a chain of cells comprising the sensory pathways (Gardner & Martin, 2000). In the case of the auditory system, these receptors are predominantly inner hair cells. These ascending pathways are serially organized from first-order neurons to higher-order neurons. Processing in the relay nuclei determines which input signals will be transmitted to the cortex. The convergent connections in these relay nuclei allow the higher-order neurons to interpret the incoming information in the context of the neighboring input activity. Noise or random activity is filtered out, while stronger sequences of repetitive activity are transmitted "upstream."

Sensory receptors have uniformly excitatory receptive fields (Gardner & Martin, 2000). Higher-order (more central) sensory pathway neurons, however, have receptive fields with both excitatory and inhibitory inputs. It is this combination of excitatory and inhibitory synapses that allows the transmission of some signals to higher centers, while inhibiting or suppressing the "noise" of surrounding, less relevant inputs. Inhibitory inputs to surrounding regions are produced by inhibitory interneurons stimulated by the dominant signal being transmitted along distinct pathways (Figure 3-1). The inhibition produced by these interneurons allows only certain signals to pass through the relay nucleus, while others are

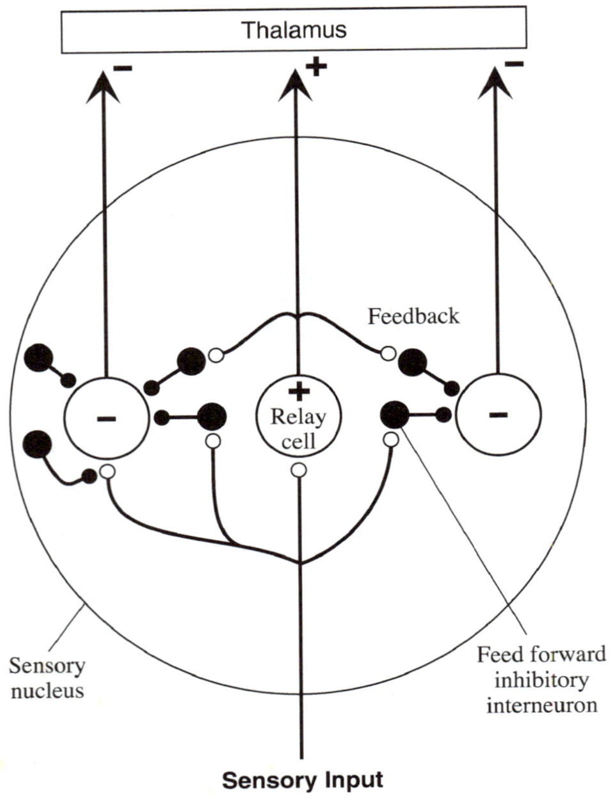

FIGURE 3–1. Example of lateral inhibition in neural pathways. Ascending excitatory signals activate local interneurons that inhibit surrounding neurons. The effect is that the dominant signal is transmitted while surrounding signals are suppressed. Adapted from *Principles of Neural Science* (p. 369), by E. R. Kandel, J. H. Schwartz, and T. M. Jessell, 1991, New York: Elsevier. Copyright 1991 by Elsevier Science Publishing Company, Inc. Adapted with permission.

blocked. The most important pathway involved in this process is the one in which inhibitory interneurons directly synapse on adjacent ascending fibers that are in close proximity to each other. Through this mechanism, the most active fiber will reduce the output of nearby fibers. This mechanism is called lateral inhibition. Higher brain centers also can send descending projections to activate inhibitory interneurons in relay centers. The combined effect of these inhibitory actions is that zones of contrasting activity are created in which a zone of more active neurons is surrounded by a zone of less active neurons. Only sensory input from the more active neurons passes through the relay nucleus.

The Reticular Formation

The reticular formation is a diffuse network of neurons that extends from the spinal cord through the core of the brainstem and into the thalamus (Vander et al., 1990) (Figure 3–2). It has a reticulated (netlike) appearance that contrasts with circumscribed nuclei in the brainstem. This appearance reflects its function—it attends to tasks that involve the entire nervous system, including arousal level, direction of attention, and awareness (all elements of consciousness). The reticular formation continuously monitors sensory information entering the CNS, and in turn exerts its influence over all regions of the CNS.

In spite of its diffuse appearance, the reticular formation is complexly organized into several subdivisions that differ in both structure and function (Brodal, 2004). In general, however, the column of neurons that comprises the reticular formation contains a medial division and a lateral division. The medial division sends out numerous long axons (efferent output) in both ascending and descending directions. These efferent projections modulate the actions of neurons involved in many functions, including autonomic activity and arousal (Saper, 2000b). The lateral division receives (afferent) input from various sensory receptors.

Another general feature of the reticular formation is that collateral fibers project perpendicularly (transversely) from the long efferent fibers, thus ensuring that these neurons cross-connect with many functionally diverse nuclei throughout the brainstem. These connections enable the reticular formation to modulate the activity of the different sensory and motor systems that are controlled by these cell groups.

Input to the Reticular Formation

The reticular formation receives and integrates signals from all types of sensory receptors (Brodal, 2004). Thus, stimulation of any receptor activates neurons in the reticular formation. For example, auditory signals reach the reticular formation via collaterals that project from ascending fibers of the auditory pathways. In addition, stimulation of the cortex, hypothalamus, and limbic structures (notably the amygdala) evokes

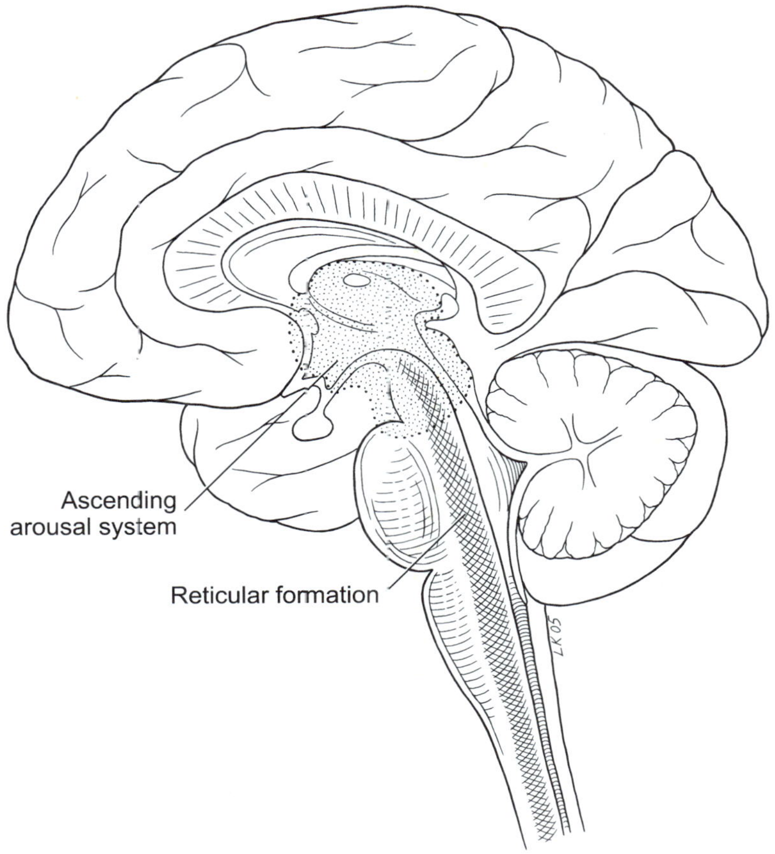

FIGURE 3–2. Areas of the reticular formation and the ascending arousal system.

activity in the reticular formation. The constant input to the reticular formation keeps it in a state of tonic activity, the level of which depends on the amount of information being received. This tonic activity is necessary to enable conscious awareness of sensory stimuli and to facilitate appropriate behavioral responses.

Reticular Formation Output to CNS

Nerve fibers of the reticular formation branch to virtually all parts of the brain and spinal cord, causing nonspecific and extremely widespread effects. These fibers exert their greatest influence on certain regions through which sensory input is modulated, including the thalamus and brainstem nuclei (Brodal, 2004). The reticular formation participates in the control of wakefulness and vigilance, as well as responsiveness to sensory stimuli by the thalamus and cortex (Saper, 2000a). Responsiveness to sensory stimuli describes the state of arousal, and requires the thalamus and cortex to be activated in such a way that they can appropriately process incoming sensory information.

Ascending Arousal System

The reticular formation is part of a system of ascending pathways, known as the ascending arousal system, that also includes the thalamus, hypothalamus, and other cell groups (Saper, 2000a) (Figure 3–2). The ascending arousal system has two major branches. One branch enters the thalamus and modulates sensory signals on their way to the cortex. The second branch has diffuse connections with the cerebral cortex via the hypothalamus. Consciousness is impaired when there is damage to either of these two branches.

Locus Coeruleus

The locus coeruleus is strongly implicated as mediating directed attention and is the primary neural center for maintaining vigilance and responsiveness to unexpected environmental stimuli (Saper, 2000a). The locus coeruleus is located in the pons and is often considered to be part of the reticular formation (Brodal, 2004). Neurons from the locus coeruleus project extensively to cortical areas, as well as to many other parts of the CNS. Its ascending projections determine which brain area will gain temporary dominance in the ongoing stream of consciousness (Vander et al., 1990). Neural activity in the locus coeruleus increases with sensory stimulation and with increased attention. When activated, these neurons release the neurotransmitter norepinephrine, which decreases background electrical activity in the brain. In this way, weak signals are suppressed and more vigorous signals are enhanced—effectively improving the signal-to-noise ratio so that sensory signals are given more prominence.

Arousal As Measured by Electroencephalography

The electroencephalogram (EEG) assesses the electrical activity of the cerebral cortex, which correlates with the level of arousal. The different waves seen in the EEG depend on the coordination, or synchronization, of cortical activity (Brodal, 2004). The general rule is that synchronization is an inverse function of arousal; that is, as arousal increases, synchronization decreases. With increased attention and alertness (i.e., increased arousal), the EEG waves become faster, smaller, and more irregular (desynchronized). The EEG waveform can detect differences between awake states (alert vs. drowsy) and between sleep states (four characteristic stages of slow wave sleep vs. rapid-eye-movement/REM sleep).

A number of experiments have confirmed that the reticular formation is responsible for determining the level of wakeful consciousness (Brodal, 2004). Unconsciousness is associated with a marked reduction in reticular formation activity, and even a small lesion in the reticular formation can cause unconsciousness. The level of arousal is controlled by reticular formation connections in the thalamus, which then project to the cortex (thalamocortical system) (Saper, 2000a). The waveform pattern seen in the EEG is thus a direct reflection of excitatory activity in the thalamocortical system.

Control of Sensory Input to Cortex

The thalamocortical system of neurons has the unique property of generating action potentials in two different patterns or modes (Saper, 2000a). In the *transmission* mode (associated with arousal), the thalamic relay neurons have a resting membrane potential that is near the firing threshold. In this mode, incoming signals cause these neurons to fire in patterns reflecting the sensory input. In the *burst* mode (associated with drowsiness), these same neurons are hyperpolarized (made less sensitive) by inhibitory input, which would cause them to not transmit incoming sensory signals to the cortex. These different functional states thus control the gating of sensory signals between the thalamus and the cortex.

Gating of Auditory Signals

Reticular formation inhibition of irrelevant signals coordinates with the thalamocortical system and other neural mechanisms to facilitate focused attention on specific stimuli or thoughts (Brodal, 2004). The combined result of these mechanisms is to restrict awareness to certain stimuli, which can only be accomplished if irrelevant stimuli are blocked from entering consciousness. The transmission of auditory and other information is largely controlled by the reticular formation. Auditory signals reach the reticular formation by collaterals of the ascending fibers in the auditory pathways. The reticular formation plays an important role in the blockage of auditory signals that are deemed irrelevant, so that only relevant signals enter consciousness. Thus, when listening to one sound, the reticular formation assists in suppressing incoming signals from other competing sounds.

Descending Control of the Auditory Pathways

There is inhibitory control of auditory impulses at all levels from the cochlea to the cortex (Brodal, 2004). More than any other sensory system, the auditory system is capable of filtering incoming information so that only certain signals reach consciousness. This selective suppression is necessary to select and attend to relevant sounds rather than irrelevant sounds. This is demonstrated by the ability to attend to a single conversation in the midst of multiple conversations.

Habituation and the Reticular Formation

The reticular formation may be at least partially responsible for habituation to sounds. Damage to the mesencephalic reticular formation in rats prevented their long-term habituation to the acoustic startle response (Jordan & Leaton, 1983). Furthermore, lesions to this area were shown to abolish previously acquired habituation to the acoustic startle response (Jordan, 1989). This form of habituation appears to be mediated by neural circuits extrinsic to the reflex circuit of the startle response. The mechanism involves accrual of increased activity within this extrinsic circuit, but the synaptic inhibitory mechanism causing habituation is not known. The mesencephalic reticular formation is a necessary link in this pathway, but there may also be other structures involved. The startle response is an excellent example of a sound-induced reaction. Habituation of a startle response represents habituation of reaction, and not of perception.

DIRECTED ATTENTION AND TINNITUS

Sensory signals are processed constantly by the brain to determine their relevance and to direct them or terminate them, as appropriate. For the person bothered by tinnitus, the tinnitus-related neural signal has been conditioned to trigger a reaction (thoughts, events, or experiences that are associated with the tinnitus) under certain circumstances. Because the tinnitus neural signal is incorrectly identified as a relevant stimulus, the signal also inappropriately receives focused attention. The filtering and blocking of irrelevant stimuli that are normally accomplished by the reticular formation and other neural mechanisms allow transmission of the tinnitus signal into cortical areas of consciousness and to the limbic and autonomic nervous systems. It is this mechanism that TRT attempts to "retrain" so that the tinnitus signal is appropriately diminished prior to entering these areas of the brain. When retraining is successful, the reactions to tinnitus are habituated. Habituation of reactions will automatically result in habituation of perception. Thus, retraining results in the tinnitus signal being *correctly* identified as an *irrelevant* stimulus, and, as such, the tinnitus does not normally evoke reactions and enter consciousness.

This chapter has focused on cognitive aspects of brain function relevant to tinnitus. For the majority of people who experience tinnitus but who are not particularly bothered by it, tinnitus is processed as an auditory signal that is essentially meaningless and thus naturally and easily habituated. For the smaller percentage who are significantly bothered by their tinnitus, emotional reactions leading to an increase in autonomic nervous system activity become the dominant factor. While emotions are significant, it is the associated reactions of the sympathetic part of the autonomic nervous system that cause tinnitus to become a clinically significant condition. Some patients have limited emotional responses but very strong autonomic responses. At the behavioral level, these patients frequently have a high level of anxiety, depression, and possibly obsessive-compulsive tendencies or disorders (Erlandsson, 2000).

4

Emotions

The *Random House College Dictionary* provides a definition of emotion that is befitting TRT:

> an affective state of consciousness in which joy, sorrow, fear, hate, or the like, is experienced, as distinguished from cognitive and volitional states of consciousness; usually accompanied by certain physiological changes, as increased heartbeat, respiration, or the like, and often overt manifestations, as crying, shaking, or laughing.

It is important to note from this definition that there are two components to an emotion: its characteristic physical sensation and conscious awareness of the physical sensation (Iversen, Kupfermann, & Kandel, 2000). With respect to TRT, conscious awareness of the physical sensation may be present, but it is not a necessary aspect of the tinnitus clinical condition.

An understanding of how emotions are represented in the brain is important to understand the neurophysiological model of tinnitus that is the basis for TRT. There are a number of relevant issues: (a) some stimuli acquire emotional significance; (b) autonomic responses are triggered by stimuli that have emotional significance; (c) there are distinct neural circuits within the brain for both conscious and subconscious aspects of emotion; and (d) an emotional response involves interaction between conscious and subconscious components (Iversen, Kupfermann, et al. 2000).

THEORIES OF EMOTIONS

Various theories of emotions have evolved over the years, as reviewed by Iversen, Kupfermann, et al. (2000) and by LeDoux (1998). Each theory has attempted to explain what happens between an event (or stimulus) that causes a conscious emotional feeling, and the feeling itself. The traditional view was that an emotional stimulus would first produce conscious awareness, which would then activate the appropriate physical response. This view was later replaced by the opposite theory, i.e., that conscious awareness of an emotional state follows the physical emotional response. The latest understanding is that an emotion-evoking stimulus is evaluated initially at the subconscious level. If conditioned reflexes are involved, this subconscious evaluation is followed by a tendency to respond in a predetermined way, and then by the emotional response itself. Finally, conscious experience of the emotion follows this chain of events. This theory is supported by the observation that physical emotional reactions can occur even to situations that do not reach conscious awareness (i.e., to subconscious stimuli). Thus, subconscious processing can produce physical emotional states independent of any conscious thought. This is the basis for the implementation of TRT. Tinnitus patients need to understand that their emotional state is partially affected by subconscious reactions.

NEURAL CIRCUITRY OF EMOTIONS

Neural mechanisms of emotions involve both cortical and subcortical components (Iversen, Kupfermann, et al., 2000). The cortical component evaluates emotions at the conscious and subconscious levels and involves the cerebral cortex, particularly the cingulate cortex and prefrontal cortex. The subcortical component involves the hypothalamus, which controls physical emotional responses. The amygdala is vital for coordinating activities between these cortical and subcortical processes of emotions. These structures, along with many others involved with emotions, have been referred to collectively as the *limbic system*. The limbic system, in turn, exercises control over the autonomic nervous system.

Clinically significant tinnitus is defined by the negative autonomic and emotional reactions that it causes. To be clear, these negative emotional reactions are "physiological changes," as indicated in the definition of emotion at the start of this chapter. Physiological changes that are associated with emotions describe precisely the reactions induced by the sympathetic part of the autonomic nervous system (see Chapter 5). Controlling these negative reactions is the main objective of most methods of tinnitus treatment, including TRT. With TRT, however, the task is approached from the perspective of modifying the underlying neurophysiological processes. The intent is to elucidate the neural circuitry that causes the reactions, and to provide treatment designed to modify the activity in this circuitry in a manner that mitigates the reactions. It is important to understand that these reactions are only indirectly caused by the limbic system. While the limbic and autonomic nervous systems are closely linked, the two systems are anatomically and functionally separate.

The Fear System of the Brain

To understand the neurophysiological and psychological consequences of tinnitus, it is helpful to understand the fear system of the brain. LeDoux (1998, p. 128) explains that the fear system does much more than cause the experience of fear: "It is a system that detects danger and produces responses that maximize the probability of surviving a dangerous situation in the most beneficial way. In other words, it is a system of defensive behavior." The concept of fear involves a broad range of negative emotional states: "alarm, scare, worry, concern, misgiving, qualm, disquiet, uneasiness, wariness, nervousness, edginess, jitteriness, apprehension, anxiety, trepidation, fright, dread, anguish, panic, terror, horror, consternation, distress, unnerved, distraught, threatened, defensive" (p. 129). Each of these terms is relevant to clinically significant tinnitus, and each involves the neural circuitry of fear.

The simplest way to understand the fear system is to think of the amygdala as the hub of the system (LeDoux, 1998). In essence, the amygdala uses input from various areas of the brain to evaluate the potential need for defensive behavior. The amygdala in turn projects to other brain areas to direct specific responses. The most important of these is the hypothalamus, which exerts control over the entire autonomic nervous system. Thus, the fear response is mediated predominantly through the amygdala-hypothalamus axis. Further components of the fear system are covered in the remainder of this chapter.

LIMBIC SYSTEM

In the early 1950s it was theorized that the limbic system concept offered a conclusive explanation of the neural mechanisms of emotions (LeDoux, 2000; MacLean, 1949, 1952). Since then it has been commonly accepted that limbic brain structures underlie emotions and subconscious processes, in contrast to the cortex, which mediates conscious activity (Brodal, 2004). Specific brain structures have been identified that define the limbic system, but most of these structures are now known to participate in a number of other functional processes that are gradually being clarified. It is therefore apparent that the limbic system does not function as a distinct or stand-alone system. LeDoux (1998) has summarized the concerns: (a) there is no agreement as to which brain structures actually constitute the limbic system; (b) the hypothalamus was previously thought to connect only to the limbic system, but recent discoveries have shown that it connects to all levels of the brain, including the neocortex (outer cortical layer); (c) the limbic system was thought to be defined on the basis of its involvement in regulating the autonomic nervous system, but it is now known that some limbic areas are actually involved more in other functions (e.g., the hippocampus is involved mostly in cognition); and (d) areas not considered part of the limbic system are now known to exert control primarily over autonomic function.

For the reasons listed above, there is little evidence for the existence of an anatomically distinct limbic system. The limbic system as a functional concept, however, is an important and useful component of the TRT counseling protocol (P. J. Jastreboff & M. M. Jastreboff, 2003) for facilitating the presentation of complex neurophysiological concepts to patients. Although this may seem to present a conflict, we adhere to the following view: Use of the term *limbic system*, although technically inaccurate, does indicate correctly that there are certain brain structures that mediate emotions. In fact, the term has come into common usage to refer to the emotional brain and it continues to be used in lectures and books. We therefore do not propose to abandon the concept, as advocated by LeDoux (1998). Rather, the concept can be used with the caveat that the limbic system is a loosely defined physiological system. A precise definition of the limbic system, or its anatomic delineation, is not needed for either the neurophysiological model of tinnitus or for TRT.

Brain regions that are usually mentioned as being part of the limbic system include the cingulate gyrus, entorhinal area, hippocampus, and amygdala (Brodal, 2004) (Figure 4-1). In addition, certain cortical structures are involved in the processing of emotions, particularly the prefrontal cortex and the insula. There are further dense interconnections between a deep region of the brain, referred to as the basal forebrain (including the nucleus accumbens), and both limbic structures and cortical areas. These connections indicate involvement of the basal forebrain with both cognitive and emotional processes.

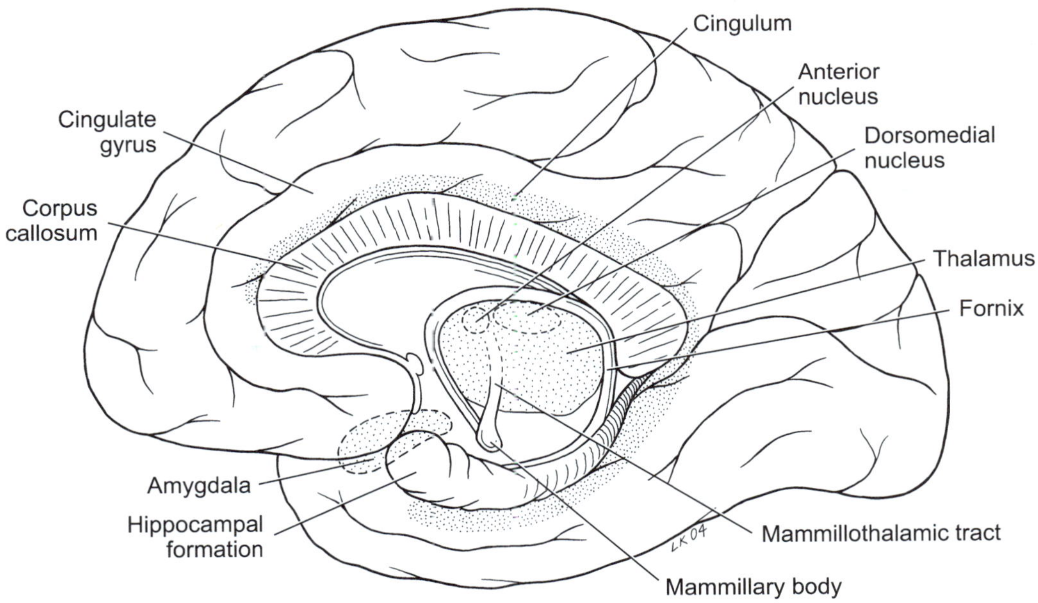

FIGURE 4–1. Diagrammatic medial view of the brain diencephalon and cortex showing regions that are commonly associated with the limbic system (stippled areas). The predominant limbic structures include the cingulate gyrus, hippocampal formation, amygdala, and entorhinal area. (The entorhinal area is not labeled—it is superficial to the hippocampus and posterior to the amygdala.)

It appears the processing of emotions does not involve a specific center that corresponds with each emotion. Emotional responses, as well as all behavioral reactions, involve many areas of the brain, including the amygdala, reticular formation, hippocampal region, septal area, large regions of the cortex, and parts of the hypothalamus. As a general rule, brain functions that are more complex involve broader distributions of neural networks to perform the necessary processing.

Hypothalamus

There are multiple nuclear regions within the hypothalamus that work in a coordinated manner to control all autonomic and somatic responses (Iversen, Kupfermann, et al., 2000). The limbic system interprets the emotional meanings of an external stimulus (for example, whether threatening or friendly) and routes that information to the hypothalamus (Vander, Sherman, & Luciano, 1990). The hypothalamus then integrates the endocrine, autonomic, and some of the motor activities to enact an emotional behavior in response to the stimulus. The elicited emotions should be appropriate to the situation but often they are not.

Amygdala

The most important structure of the limbic system is the amygdala, which coordinates the activity of the hypothalamus and the cortical limbic areas (cingulate cortex and parahippocampal gyrus) (Iversen, Kupfermann, et al., 2000). The amygdala thus performs the central role of controlling both the physical expression and the conscious awareness of emotions.

As auditory signals travel bilaterally through the medial geniculate nuclei of the thalamus, this information is conveyed directly and rapidly to the lateral amygdala, which mediates emotional responses (Iversen, Kupfermann, et al., 2000; LeDoux, 1992; LeDoux et al., 1987). The lateral nucleus of the amygdala receives the input, and output is via the central nucleus of the amygdala. Acoustic information from the thalamus and the auditory cortex converges in the lateral nucleus, the former signal being a rapid and rudimentary code and the latter a slower, more detailed message (LeDoux, 1998). Emotional processing may depend on this interaction between thalamic and cortical auditory stimuli converging in the amygdala (Figure 4–2). The dual outputs from the central amygdala ultimately trigger autonomic changes and behavioral fear responses via two separate pathways, respectively, the (a) lateral hypothalamic, brainstem, and spinal premotor neurons of the autonomic nervous system and (b) midbrain central gray matter. Fear conditioning is mediated via a direct thalamo-amygdala projection independent of the cortical auditory pathways (Hu, 2003; LeDoux, 1992; LeDoux, Iwata, Cicchetti, & Reis, 1988; Mahlke & Wallhausser-

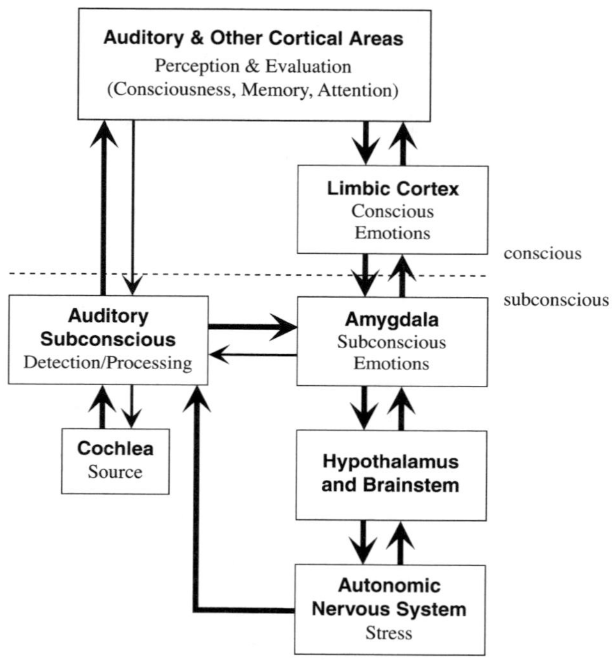

FIGURE 4–2. TRT neurophysiological model of tinnitus (P. J. Jastreboff & Hazell, 2004). The auditory areas of the model are on the left. The other areas of the model (limbic and autonomic nervous systems) are nonauditory areas of the brain (right side) that are thought to be involved when tinnitus is problematic. Adapted from *Tinnitus Retraining Therapy: Implementing the Neurophysiological Model* (p. 35) by P. J. Jastreboff and J. W. P. Hazell, 2004, New York: Cambridge University Press. Copyright 2004 by Cambridge University Press. Adapted with permission from the author.

Franke, 2004; Wallhausser-Franke et al., 2003; Zhang, Kaltenbach, Wang, & Kim, 2003). This is a key neural pathway in the TRT neurophysiological model.

The information conveyed in this manner may be especially important in initiating rapid emotional responses to immediate danger and may further prepare the amygdala to receive later information from cortical centers that have undergone greater processing. Stimulation of the projections to the amygdala from both the thalamus and the cortex produces long-term synaptic changes in the amygdala, which is a process underlying emotional learning (LeDoux, 2000). Sounds that do not normally elicit an emotional reaction can be paired with a threatening stimulus so that the previously neutral sound will by itself evoke an emotional response, such as anxiety. In other words, a conditioned reflex is created. Conversely, if a threatening stimulus is paired repeatedly with a neutral sound, the threatening stimulus can acquire emotional neutrality. This latter concept is called habituation of reactions, or passive extinction of conditioned reflexes, and is the basis for the crucial use of sound therapy with TRT (P. J. Jastreboff & M. M. Jastreboff, 2003).

EMOTION VERSUS COGNITION

Although everyone knows implicitly what an emotion is, researchers have been unable to agree on its precise definition (LeDoux, 1998). What is necessary for TRT, however, is not to define emotions, but to understand how emotions are processed by the nervous system. The TRT neurophysiological model (Figure 4-2) provides a framework for this. The model also makes distinctions between emotional and cognitive processing. Furthermore, there are critical TRT issues that relate to subconscious versus conscious aspects of both emotions and cognitions. These various distinctions need to be understood unambiguously by the clinician to effectively explain the model in the clearest terms to patients. For purposes of our discussion, emotion refers to passion or feeling, while cognition refers to reason, intellect, or verbal thinking. As already mentioned, emotions have the two components of physiological reactions and cognitive awareness of the reactions.

On the physiological level, emotions are essentially automatic reactions to significant events that do not require conscious awareness (LeDoux, 1998). This is again a description of conditioned reflexes that are essential to understanding the TRT neurophysiological model. Emotions are, of course, more than just reflexive physiological responses. Consciousness has a role in emotions, producing subjective emotional experiences, or "emotional feelings" (depicted in Figure 4-2 as descending arrows from the cortex to the limbic and autonomic nervous systems in the model). When we become consciously aware of, for example, activation of the body's defensive system, we "feel afraid." When exposed to an emotionally significant stimulus, the stimulus causes both a physiological response and a conscious emotional feeling.

It bears repeating that the limbic system has been accepted as the predominant neural basis for emotion for over 50 years. This viewpoint has been compatible with the observation that higher-level cognitive processes occur only in mammals that are exclusively endowed with a neocortex (LeDoux, 2000). Humans have the greatest cognitive abilities, which correspond with their maximum amount of neocortical tissue. Not all researchers, however, agree with the clear delineation between the limbic system and the neocortex as mediators of emotions and cognition, respectively. LeDoux (2000) points out that as early as the mid-1950s it was discovered that the hippocampus, which was then considered the central limbic coordinating center, was critical to the formation of long-term memories. Since long-term memory is a distinctly cognitive function, this discovery contradicted the concept that "primitive" limbic structures subserve only emotional activity. Since that time, definition of the limbic system has been a "moving target." There is still no agreement as to the criteria that would determine which brain areas are parts of the limbic system. Further, there is little understanding as to how emotions are produced by the limbic system. In spite of these issues, there is abundant evidence that limbic areas do play a role in emotions, and that there are cognitive functions that are processed independent of the limbic system.

EMOTIONS AND TINNITUS

Brain mechanisms are constantly at work monitoring all sounds for their meaning. Most sounds are interpreted as meaningless and are quickly habituated (Domjan & Burkhard, 1986). For other sounds, meaning is attached, and these sounds (including tinnitus) can evoke strong emotional reactions (Hazell, 1999; Iversen, Kupfermann, et al., 2000). This link between emotion and sound may be the basis for psychological distress in the approximately 20% of people in whom permanent tinnitus manifests a clinically significant condition (A. Davis & Refaie, 2000; P. J. Jastreboff, Gray, & Gold, 1996; P. J. Jastreboff & Hazell, 1998). If the tinnitus receives extended focused attention, the individual may enter a "vicious circle" of progressively increasing anxiety associated with the conscious perception of tinnitus (P. J. Jastreboff et al., 1996; P. J. Jastreboff & Hazell, 1998). The vicious circle may also be associated with depression and/or obsessive-compulsive tendencies.

The two issues that must be addressed clinically for problematic tinnitus are inappropriately heightened attention to the tinnitus and the associated emotional reactions. The TRT protocol is designed to promote long-term habituation of tinnitus-induced reactions, and subsequently habituation of the tinnitus perception. TRT counseling is aimed at reclassification of tinnitus to the category of an emotionally neutral stimulus, which is important to initiate and sustain the process of habituation. The role of sound therapy is to decrease the relative strength of the tinnitus-related neural activity in the nervous system by increasing the level of background neural activity. Sound therapy decreases the tinnitus-signal-to-background-noise ratio, which facilitates habituation of the tinnitus signal (J. A. Henry, Schechter, Nagler, & Fausti, 2002; P. J. Jastreboff, 1996, 2000; P. J. Jastreboff et al., 1996; P. J. Jastreboff & Hazell, 1998, 2004). Appropriate implementation of sound therapy is a critical element of TRT.

The fear system of the brain was described above as mediating a broad range of negative emotional states. It is important to understand this fear reaction system to clarify how tinnitus can directly affect emotional responses. A simplified approach is to consider the basic neural routing of sensory information that activates the fear system. All sensory stimuli (except olfactory) activate pathways that travel through the thalamus. In order for sensory stimuli to cause an emotional response, they must activate emotional memories stored in the amygdala. From the thalamus there are two parallel routes that the information can follow to reach the amygdala. LeDoux (1998) refers to these two routes as the "low road" and the "high road" (Figure 4-3). The low road is a direct connection from the thalamus to the amygdala. The high road is a parallel route from the thalamus to the sensory cortex to the amygdala. Sensory information travels through the low road to enable the quickest possible response to threatening stimuli. This direct information lacks cortical processing and thus provides only a crude representation of the stimulus. However, it does facilitate a fear reaction even before there is conscious awareness of the stimulus, which may provide the critical difference in surviving a dangerous situation. The same information that travels the high road requires additional links, and thus additional time, but it has

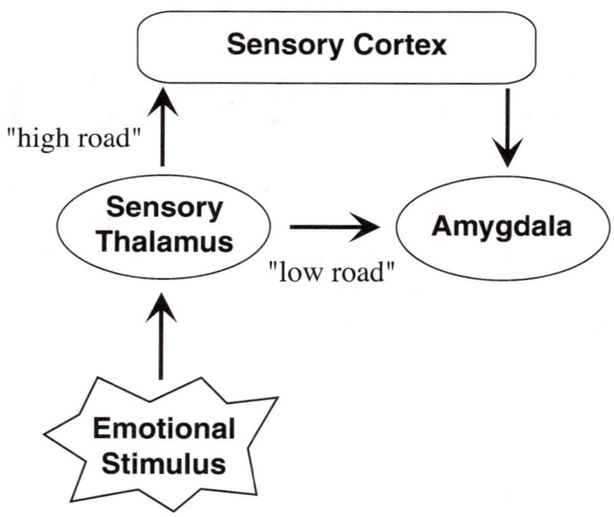

FIGURE 4–3. Routing of neural signals for emotionally significant information (LeDoux, 1998). The subconscious route goes directly from the sensory thalamus to the amygdala ("low road"). The conscious (indirect) route travels first to the sensory cortex ("high road"). Adapted from *The Emotional Brain* (p. 164) by J. E. LeDoux, 1998, New York: Touchstone. Copyright 1998 by Simon & Schuster. Adapted with permission from the publisher.

the advantage of cortical processing to discriminate the stimulus and to evaluate its potential for danger. The indirect cortical pathway also is able to override the direct thalamic pathway, which serves to prevent inappropriate responses.

Although the neural site of tinnitus generation cannot be determined, P. J. Jastreboff's neurophysiological model assumes, for didactic purposes, that the signal is generated in the cochlea in the majority of cases (according to his "discordant damage/dysfunction" theory of tinnitus generation) (P. J. Jastreboff, 1990, 1995; Kaltenbach et al., 1998). (Note that according to the neurophysiological model the tinnitus signal can be generated at any level of the auditory system.) The cause of the tinnitus signal is irrelevant from the point of view of the neurophysiological model of tinnitus and for TRT. There is only the need to depict a neural correlate of tinnitus. In this respect there is consensus that some tinnitus-related activity is generated within the auditory pathways, such as the dorsal cochlear nucleus, auditory nerve fibers, inferior colliculi, thalamus, or primary and secondary auditory cortices. Experimental data support this postulate (Bauer, 2004; Chen & P. J. Jastreboff, 1995; Eggermont & Roberts, 2004; P. J. Jastreboff, Hansen, P. G. Sasaki, & C. T. Sasaki, 1986; Kaltenbach, 2000, 2006; Kaltenbach et al., 1998; Lockwood, Burkard, & Salvi, 2004; Lockwood et al., 1998; Reyes et al., 2002).

Acoustic signals from a damaged cochlea result in an "altered code for silence" secondary to discordant damage between outer and inner hair cells. These signals ascend the auditory pathways through the cochlear nuclei, superior olivary complex, lateral lemniscus, inferior colliculi, and medial geniculate nuclei (Cacace, 2003; Mahlke & Wallhausser-Franke, 2004) (see Figure 1-4). Assuming a cochlear origin, the tinnitus neural signal would not simply take this direct route from the cochlea to the auditory cortex. Rather, there is an early exit along the ascending auditory pathways that leads to a "shortcut route" to potential fear, anxiety, and stress responses. This shortcut route is LeDoux's (1998) low road from the auditory thalamus (medial geniculate) to the lateral amygdala (Figure 4-3). From the medial geniculate nuclei, these signals diverge to follow the low and the high roads to the amygdala. Via the low road, signals pass directly to the lateral nucleus of the amygdala. If these direct signals carry emotional significance, they proceed via the central output nuclei of the amygdala to elicit autonomic and behavioral fear responses via the hypothalamus, brainstem, and spinal premotor neurons of the autonomic nervous system and the midbrain central gray (Hu, 2003; Mahlke & Wallhausser-Franke, 2004; Wallhausser-Franke et al., 2003; Zhang et al., 2003).

Auditory signals are continually monitored by the amygdala via both conscious and unconscious routes. The amygdala detects whether a signal has emotional significance. If not, then the signal is blocked from transmission to the hypothalamus and autonomic nervous system. Emotionally significant stimuli, however, are routed to these areas to effect fear and other emotional responses (that may or may not be appropriate). This routing of auditory signals is the essence of the TRT neurophysiological model of tinnitus (Figure 4-2). The low road and high road, as described by LeDoux (1998), are represented by the low (subconscious or subcortical) and high (conscious or cortical) loop, respectively, in the neurophysiological model (P. J. Jastreboff, 2000). Perhaps the most important component in the model is the direct, subconscious route for the tinnitus signal to activate the amygdala.

Chronic tinnitus is a constant signal, but it does not always activate the cortical loop; i.e., tinnitus does not enter consciousness 100% of the time. However, the signal is continually active at the subconscious level, which causes constant monitoring by the amygdala. If the tinnitus has emotional significance, then the amygdala responds accordingly (and inappropriately) to activate a variety of autonomic responses, including the stress response. The subconscious loop shown in the neurophysiological model must therefore be addressed in any program of therapy for tinnitus. TRT uses a structured program of counseling as the primary method to reclassify tinnitus to the category of a neutral stimulus. Reclassification of tinnitus to a neutral stimulus must be accomplished in order to achieve habituation of both perception and reaction to tinnitus.

5

Stress

The physical effects of severe tinnitus are best understood in the context of the stress response. This also incorporates the concepts of physiologic homeostasis and of the autonomic nervous system with its sympathetic and parasympathetic divisions. The stress reaction of TRT has been referred to as the fight-or-flight response, which is an emergency reaction triggered by intense emotion (Iversen, Kupfermann et al., 2000). However, stress does not necessarily progress to the level of the fight-or-flight response. Stress should be thought of as a constellation of physiological responses on a continuum of intensity, with fight-or-flight being the extreme of these combined responses. Thus, the fight-or-flight response is not a critical aspect of TRT, although it is a well-understood reaction that helps to explain some of the stress concepts during TRT counseling.

HOMEOSTASIS

Homeostasis refers to constancy of the body's internal environment. This constancy is maintained through physiological mechanisms that function primarily to regulate the fluids that bathe our cells (Carlson, 1991). The hypothalamus is the principal site for controlling both neural and endocrine functions that maintain homeostasis (Vander et al., 1990). Thus, the hypothalamus is the single most important brain area for regulating the internal milieu of the body.

SOMATIC VERSUS AUTONOMIC NERVOUS SYSTEMS

The human nervous system can be viewed as two semi-independent systems (Wilson-Pauwels, Stewart, & Akesson, 1997). First, the somatic nervous system enables interaction with the external environment, using input from the senses and producing output in the form of voluntary behavioral responses. Activities mediated by the somatic nervous system, such as hearing, tactile sensation, and movement, can be consciously perceived or controlled. Second, the autonomic nervous system controls the body's internal environment by maintaining homeostasis. Unlike the somatic nervous system, there is generally no conscious awareness of the underlying neural activities that take place within the autonomic nervous system. The manifestations of this neural activity may be observed (heart rate, sweating, etc.), but they are involuntary and normally uncontrollable.

The somatic and autonomic nervous systems are organized in a similar fashion (Wilson-Pauwels et al., 1997). Both are activated by sensory neurons from the body's periphery and from higher levels of the nervous system. These input signals are transmitted to interneurons that process the information and direct appropriate responses through motor neurons to effector cells.

Whereas somatic motor neurons activate skeletal muscle fibers exclusively, autonomic motor neurons have multiple targets: smooth muscle, cardiac muscle, secretory (glandular) cells, and chromaffin cells in the adrenal medulla (Wilson-Pauwels et al., 1997). The somatic and autonomic nervous systems differ mainly in how they control their respective responses. The somatic nervous system controls voluntary muscular activity via direct connections between the CNS and skeletal muscles. The cell bodies of the motor neurons reside in specific CNS nuclei and project directly to their target cells via two-neuron pathways from motor cortex to the spinal cord, then to specific muscles. Autonomic motor neurons instead use a two-neuron chain to activate involuntary muscles: preganglionic motor neurons have cell bodies that reside in the CNS and project to postganglionic motor neurons in the autonomic ganglia, which in turn synapse in target organs. This divergent mechanism of the autonomic nervous system offers several advantages, especially the ability of large areas of the body to be influenced by few central neurons.

SYMPATHETIC AND PARASYMPATHETIC DIVISIONS OF THE AUTONOMIC NERVOUS SYSTEM

The autonomic nervous system is usually defined as consisting of sympathetic and parasympathetic divisions (Iversen, Iversen, & Saper, 2000) (Figure 5-1). (There is also the enteric division, which maintains semi-autonomous control over gastrointestinal processes.) Although these two divisions operate in conjunction with each other, their separate functions can be thought of as *fight-or-flight* for the sympathetic division, and *rest-and-digest* for the parasympathetic division. The two divisions are generally antagonistic, and they often exert opposing control over the same organs. This balance of their respective activities is what maintains body homeostasis, mediated largely through negative feedback mechanisms that act upon the hypothalamus.

FIGHT-OR-FLIGHT RESPONSE

The terms *stress* and *fight-or-flight* are often used interchangeably to refer to anything that is perceived as threatening to the maintenance of homeostasis (Brodal, 2004). Fight-or-flight, however, refers specifically to physiologic events that occur in response to one's safety being threatened (Wilson-Pauwels et al., 1997). The threat can be real or perceived; thus, the flight-or-flight response is a perception that is determined by the individual and the circumstance. When a threat is perceived, the person is mobilized to either mount a defense (fight) or escape from the threat (flight). The expectation of a threat can be as real as the threat itself, and the fight-or-flight response can be sustained in the absence of any threat.

Both fight and flight require that the body prepare itself for sudden, vigorous muscle action (Wilson-Pauwels et al., 1997). The body prepares itself for fight-or-flight in three general phases.

Phase One: Activation of Sympathetic Cascade

The amygdala receives "fear" signals that it transmits to the hypothalamus (Iversen, Kupfermann, et al., 2000). The hypothalamus in turn signals the sympathetic preganglionic neurons in the spinal cord to activate (a) the chromaffin cells in the adrenal medulla and (b) the sympathetic postganglionic neurons throughout the body (Wilson-Pauwels et al., 1997).

Phase Two: Release of Large Quantities of Sympathetic Neurotransmitters

The adrenal medulla secretes mainly adrenaline (epinephrine) into the bloodstream (Wilson-Pauwels et al., 1997). Noradrenaline (norepinephrine) is the main neurotransmitter secreted by the sympathetic postganglionic nerve endings and transmitted directly to the effector cells. Although the direct effects of adrenaline and noradrenaline on the body are essentially the same, adrenaline lasts about 10 times longer because noradrenaline is removed more rapidly from the blood.

Phase Three: Changes in Body Function Caused by Neurotransmitters

A number of body changes are caused by the release of neurotransmitters (Wilson-Pauwels et al.,

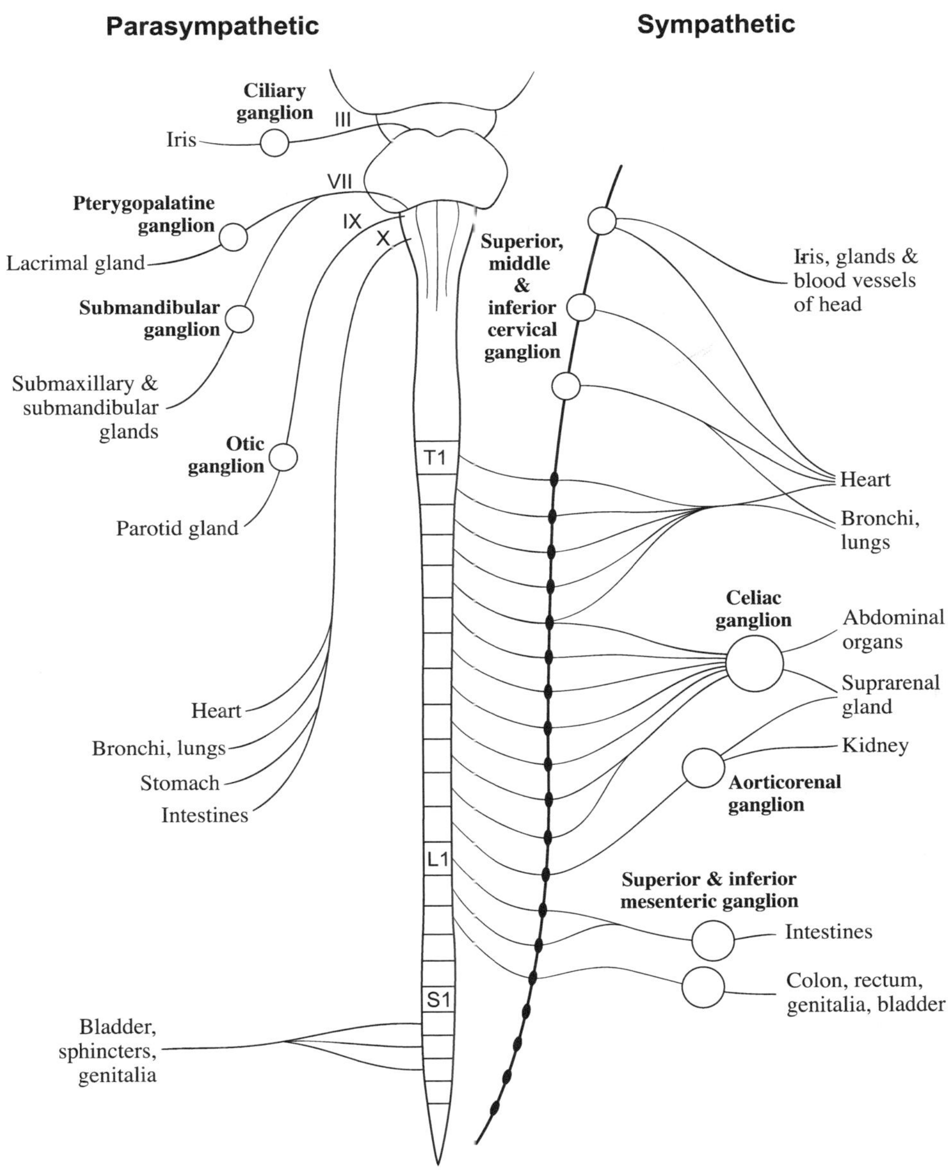

FIGURE 5–1. The autonomic nervous system, consisting of the sympathetic and parasympathetic divisions. Their opposing actions are evident by the fact both systems innervate the same organ systems. These descending outflows from the autonomic system originate in the brain and sensations from their target organs eventually feed back on the same brain areas via the ascending arousal system for modulation and control. Stress-induced autonomic outflow can lead to inappropriate activity in these organs, creating the vicious circle of neurotransmitter release, abnormal organ functions, mental problems, and even life-threatening disease.

1997). First, the muscles must be prepared for intense activity. This requires energy, which is accomplished by the breakdown of glycogen in muscles to produce glucose. Intense muscle activity also requires an increase in oxygen delivery and in carbon dioxide removal, which is accomplished by dilation of the blood vessels that course through the muscles. Second, there are changes in liver activity to facilitate release of glucose (by hepatocytes) into the circulation to be carried to muscles. Third, heart activity must increase to provide a greater blood supply to muscles. Adrenaline and noradrenaline act upon receptors in the sinoatrial (SA) node to increase heart rate, and in the atrioventricular (AV) node to slow conduction time. Cardiac output is defined as stroke volume x rate. Thus, this sequence of events increases cardiac output by increasing ventricular filling and the force of contraction (stroke volume) for each increased heartbeat (rate). Fourth, neurotransmitters dilate the bronchi in the lungs and increase the respiratory rate, both of which increase oxygen and decrease carbon dioxide in the blood. Finally, various other body changes take place, including constriction of blood vessels in the skin and viscera (which makes more blood available for the muscles) and sweating (which helps to dissipate the heat caused by additional muscle activity).

PROLONGED STRESS

As discussed in Chapter 3, stress can be viewed as a component of the ascending arousal system (see Figure 3-2). Activation of the arousal system is normally beneficial for facilitating development, learning, and adaptive behaviors (Brodal, 2004). When arousal is prolonged, however, various diseases can result. For example, recurrent fight-or-flight responses can lead to heart disease because high levels of epinephrine (adrenaline) provoke the release of fats—clogging arteries, impeding the flow of blood, and eventually damaging the heart. Heart disease caused by stress is just one of many links between health and "state of mind." Other conditions, such as ulcers and asthma, have long been considered psychosomatic illnesses that can develop in response to chronic emotional upset. It now appears that every aspect of our health can be influenced by our mental state (F. Lechin, van der Dijs, & Lechin, 2002).

STRESS PATHWAYS

It was discussed in Chapter 4 that sensory stimuli with emotional significance activate the amygdala via two pathways: the *low road* and the *high road* (LeDoux, 1998, 2000). The low road refers to direct connections between the sensory thalamus and the amygdala, while the high road refers to an indirect, longer route from the sensory thalamus to the cortex to the amygdala (see Figure 4-3). These connections, which are also depicted in the neurophysiological model of tinnitus (see Figure 4-2), now can be expanded upon to provide an overall picture of the stress pathways and their impact upon the body.

Activation of the amygdala causes a chain of reactions through the "stress axis" of the hypothalamus, pituitary gland, and adrenal cortex (Figure 5-2) (M. Davis, 2000; LeDoux, 1998). The paraventricular nucleus of the hypothalamus sends corticotrophin-releasing factor (CRF) to the pituitary gland, which releases adrenocorticotropic hormone (ACTH) into the bloodstream. This circulating ACTH causes the adrenal gland to release adrenaline. In addition to adrenaline's effects on the body (see Flight-or-Flight Response above), it also travels into the brain where it instructs the amygdala to keep activating the hypothalamus. This positive feedback loop remains in effect as long as a stressful stimulus is present. Adrenaline also acts on the hippocampus, but with an inhibitory ("slow down") message (Figure 5-2). Thus, the hippocampus and amygdala are critically involved in the balance of neural input to the hypothalamus for controlling the release of stress hormones. It is important to note that persistent stress can cause irreversible damage to the hippocampus and permanently impair memory functions (McEwen et al., 1992).

STRESS AND TINNITUS

The vicious circle of tinnitus awareness and reaction produces a sustained stress response in the body. Medical research shows clearly that such a prolonged condition can result in serious health consequences, some of which have been mentioned in this chapter. Stress has also been linked to cancer, and even to cataracts, because the circulating and intracellular antioxidants that normally protect against these conditions are used up by a sustained stress response (Abel, 1999). Stress is certainly toxic to the body and tinnitus

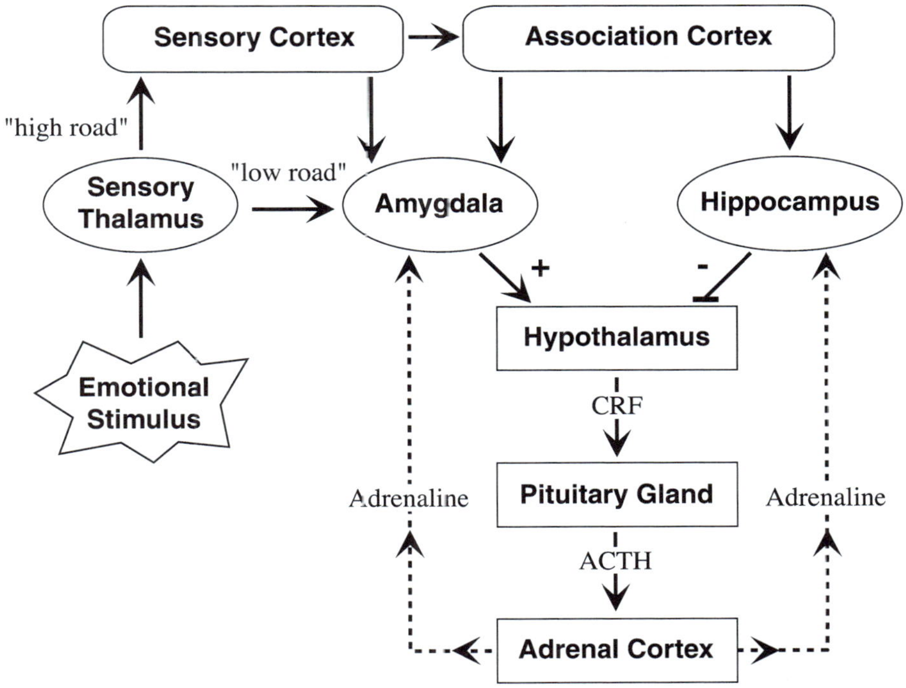

FIGURE 5–2. The stress pathways. Through these neural pathways, sensory stimuli associated with fear activate the stress response. CRF = corticotrophin-releasing factor; ACTH = adrenocorticotropic hormone. (Adapted from *The Emotional Brain: The Mysterious Underpinnings of Emotional Life* (p. 241), by J. E. LeDoux, 1998, New York: Touchstone. Copyright 1998 by Simon & Schuster, Inc. Adapted with permission from the publisher.)

is a greater stress inducer than one normally assigns to this phantom noise.

The neurophysiological model of tinnitus (see Figure 4–2) shows that tinnitus-related neural activity can ultimately activate the autonomic nervous system—specifically its sympathetic division. Activation of the autonomic nervous system results in a cascade of physiological responses, only a few of which have been mentioned in this chapter. These physiological responses include negative physiological and behavioral reactions, most of which can be considered components of the stress response. Reducing tinnitus-associated stress is a primary objective of treatment with TRT.

It is essential to understand that the tinnitus signal can activate the subconscious route (low road) shown in the neurophysiological model regardless of whether the tinnitus enters consciousness. While all sensory stimuli have this same capability, the tinnitus signal is unique in that it is continuously active. Other sensory signals occur only in response to our exposure to different environmental stimuli. Tinnitus, however, does not depend on external stimulation—it is a constant stimulus. If the tinnitus signal carries emotional significance, then it can cause sustained activation of the sympathetic division of the autonomic nervous system. Emotionally significant tinnitus thus has the capability of keeping the body in a state of chronic stress.

Stress is cumulative. We all experience stress to various degrees. The stress caused by tinnitus thus adds to any other stress that is experienced at a point in time. This overlay may have a minor additive effect, or it can be the primary contributor. It can be difficult to ascertain the degree to which tinnitus contributes to the overall stress condition of a patient due to the different psychological characteristics and life experiences that are unique to each patient. It is thus critical to perform an in-depth interview of the patient to determine the contribution of the patient's tinnitus to the overall level of stress being experienced. Furthermore, it may be that the patient's tinnitus is less of a stress inducer than other aspects of his or her life, and dealing with these other issues may reduce overall stress to the point that the contribution of tinnitus is manageable. This could influence the approach taken in helping that patient and emphasizes the need for a thorough patient evaluation.

In Chapter 10 we describe the TRT Initial Interview, which contains a series of questions designed to assess the effect of tinnitus on daily life activities. Ultimately, successful treatment will mitigate the effects of tinnitus on these activities. This can only be accomplished if the tinnitus signal is reclassified to the category of emotionally neutral stimuli. This reclassification results in a tinnitus neural signal that does not cause activity beyond the auditory system, at most reaching the amygdala. When this occurs, the patient will have habituated the reactions caused by tinnitus. The primary means of accomplishing this goal is proper counseling. The counseling is augmented by sound therapy, but sound therapy alone is normally not successful in achieving habituation to tinnitus reactions.

6

Learning and Memory

The word *retraining* in Tinnitus Retraining Therapy refers to the overall objective of TRT, which is to "retrain" the patient's brain so that the tinnitus-related neural signal becomes habituated (P. J. Jastreboff & M. M. Jastreboff, 2001). The treatment technique takes advantage of learning and memory processes that occur in the brain to distinguish meaningful versus meaningless auditory stimuli. Sounds that do not carry any informational value are normally habituated, but relevant sounds gain attention and control behavior. The brain learns to distinguish between such stimuli, and memory patterns are established that enable the brain to make these distinctions automatically. In addition to the neutral, nonthreatening sound therapy, TRT counseling contributes to the process of reversing negative responses to the tinnitus percept, thus facilitating habituation. This chapter attempts to clarify these concepts by focusing on different forms of memory and learning. Special attention is given to conditioned emotional responses, habituation, and extinction, which are the learning processes that are most relevant to tinnitus distress, and therefore to treatment with TRT.

FORMS OF MEMORY

There are two fundamentally different types of memory: memory for knowledge and memory for skills (Kandel, Kupfermann, & Iversen, 2000). Different brain networks are involved in each of these forms of memory.

Explicit Memory

Memory for knowledge is referred to as explicit, or declarative, memory and involves the deliberate, conscious recall of facts and experiences that can be reported verbally (Kandel et al., 2000). Explicit memory is stored in a distributed fashion in the medial temporal lobe of the brain, i.e., not in a circumscribed storage location. Recall of explicit memories thus involves the retrieval of bits of information from separate memory stores. Memories for facts (semantic knowledge) and experiences (episodic knowledge) are stored in separate anatomical regions. Furthermore, different aspects of these memories (e.g., animal vs. plant, living vs. nonliving, physical features, appearance, auditory features, verbal descriptions, etc.) are held in separate cortical sites. Therefore, a lesion to any one of these areas will disrupt or destroy some specific aspect of explicit memories.

Implicit Memory

Memory for "doing things" is termed implicit or nondeclarative memory (Kandel et al., 2000). Implicit memory flows automatically at a subconscious level to facilitate the performance of reflexive motor or perceptual skills. This contrasts with explicit memory that must be retrieved consciously and deliberately. Explicit memory can be easily expressed verbally, while implicit memory is difficult or impossible to express in words. Learning to play a musical instrument involves implicit memory, which is acquired through repetition over many trials.

The different forms of learning described below are different mechanisms of acquiring implicit memories (Kandel et al., 2000). Each form of learning involves different brain regions. In general, the acquisition of implicit memory utilizes primarily the amygdala and cerebellum, as well as the sensory and motor systems that process what is learned.

FORMS OF LEARNING

Scientists study implicit forms of learning by exposing animals to certain sensory experiences and observing their responses. These studies have resulted in the understanding of two major classes of learning: associative and nonassociative (Kandel et al., 2000). With *associative* learning, the animal learns to associate two stimuli (classical conditioning or stimulus-outcome learning) or a behavior and a response (operant or instrumental conditioning, or response-outcome learning). *Nonassociative* forms of learning include habituation and sensitization, which are the most fundamental changes in behavior that result from any kind of experience. With nonassociative learning, the organism learns about the properties of a stimulus through a single or repeated presentation of that stimulus.

Classical Conditioning

Most people are familiar with "Pavlov's salivating dogs," which refers to a series of experiments conducted 100 years ago by the Russian scientist Ivan P. Pavlov. These experiments demonstrated that a *meaningless* stimulus (e.g., the sound of a bell) can acquire the meaning of a separate, *meaningful* stimulus (e.g., food) through repeated pairings of the two stimuli. At the beginning of the experiment, the sound of the bell has no inherent meaning and elicits no response. After pairing the bell with food, the bell acquires the food's inherent meaning, and eventually the bell alone will elicit the same responses elicited by food. Although this is a vastly oversimplified example of classical conditioning, it demonstrates an associative form of learning through which one stimulus acquires the same meaning as another stimulus by their association.

In a classical conditioning paradigm, the meaningful stimulus is referred to as the unconditioned stimulus (UCS), while the initially meaningless stimulus is referred to as the conditioned stimulus (CS) (Table 6–1). The UCS (such as food) elicits a response (salivation), and a CS (such as a tone) can acquire the meaning of the UCS through pairing of the two stimuli. The response to a UCS is called an unconditioned response (UCR). When a CS is paired with the UCS, the response to the CS alone is a conditioned response (CR).

The two fundamental principles of classical conditioning are (a) pairing a CS with a UCS results in the acquisition of a CR and (b) repeated presentation of a CS alone results in extinction of the CR (Kehoe & Macrae, 1998). With extinction, the CS loses its ability to elicit the CR because of nonreinforcement of the CS.

Conditioned Emotional Response

The conditioned emotional response refers to a set of physiological and behavioral responses that are produced by the pairing of a previously meaningless stimulus (CS) with an aversive stimulus (UCS), such as one that produces pain (Carlson, 1991). This form of classical conditioning has particular relevance to tinnitus—through this process, tinnitus can become a meaningful stimulus that elicits undesirable responses. It is important to recognize that a conditioned reflex can be created if a benign stimulus and an aversive stimulus occur close together in time (Kehoe & Macrae, 1998). The more often the stimuli are paired, the more strongly associated they will become.

Aversive stimuli elicit a variety of both specific and nonspecific responses (Carlson, 1991). For example, applying a painful stimulus to an animal's paw elicits a *specific* defensive reflex that involves withdrawing its paw from the source of the pain. In addition, *nonspecific* responses occur, which are generally under the control of the autonomic nervous system. These "fight-or-flight" responses have been described in Chapter 5 as resulting from acute secretion of stress-related

TABLE 6–1. Classical Conditioning Terminology. Also called stimulus-outcome learning, classical conditioning requires an association between stimuli. One stimulus (unconditioned stimulus) has the innate ability to elicit a response (unconditioned response), while a second stimulus (conditioned stimulus) does not normally elicit the same response, but can be conditioned to elicit the same response (conditioned response) by establishing an association between the two stimuli.

Type of Behavior	Stimulus	Response	Examples
Unlearned/unconditioned • Behavior is innate—no learning is required for the stimulus to elicit a response	**Unconditioned stimulus (UCS)**	**Unconditioned response (UCR)**	1. Food (UCS) causes salivation (UCR) 2. Shock (UCS) causes fear (UCR)
Learned/conditioned • Behavior is not innate—prior learning is required for the stimulus to elicit a response	**Conditioned stimulus (CS)**	**Conditioned response (CR)**	Tone initially causes no response (other than orienting response) 1. If tone is paired with food, tone becomes CS that elicits salivation (CR) 2. If tone is paired with shock, tone becomes CS that elicits fear (CR)

hormones and activation of the sympathetic branch of the autonomic nervous system. Nonspecific responses involve the preparation of skeletal muscles (e.g., blood flow increase) for the intense activity that would be required for responding defensively.

If an animal learns to make a specific response to avoid contact with an aversive stimulus, the nonspecific responses will eventually disappear (Carlson, 1991). Thus, learning an appropriate reaction can reduce or eliminate the emotional responses. For example, if an animal learns to retract its paw in response to a warning stimulus to avoid receiving a painful stimulus, the fight-or-flight response will diminish. In contrast, if the painful stimulus always follows the warning stimulus, regardless of the animal's behavior, the conditioned emotional response will occur after each warning stimulus.

Emotional responses can be mediated by different neural circuits (Carlson, 1991). For example, one would react emotionally to the buzz of a wasp after being stung on several occasions. The reflexive response to a buzzing sound could be accomplished by subcortical structures without involving the auditory cortex. Perception of a complex stimulus, such as the sight of a known criminal, would require participation of the medial temporal cortex (thus involving explicit memory processes).

The role of the amygdala in coordinating emotional responses is described in Chapter 4. The amygdala is the major hub between the sensory systems and effector systems that control the various components of conditioned emotional responses (Carlson, 1991; LeDoux, 1998, 2000). Many experiments have shown that electrical stimulation of the amygdala produces defensive (fight-or-flight) reactions. In humans, electrical stimulation of the amygdala elicits feelings of fear and apprehension (Iversen, Kupfermann, et al., 2000). Bilateral ablation of the amygdala in monkeys abolishes the fear response and results in placidity, compulsive hyperorality, and hypersexuality—a behavioral condition known as the Kluver-Bucy Syndrome (Gilman & Newman, 2003; LeDoux, 1998; Victor & Ropper, 2001). It has also been shown that the amygdala is the key structure for learning a conditioned emotional response (a form of implicit memory).

The amygdala consists of approximately 10 distinct nuclear areas within the temporal lobe (Doron & LeDoux, 1999; Iversen, Kupfermann, et al., 2000; Pitkanen, 2000). One of these nuclei, the basolateral complex, receives all input regarding learned emotional states, especially fear and anxiety. The basolateral complex receives auditory information from both the thalamus and primary sensory areas of the auditory cortex (Carlson, 1991; Iversen, Kupfermann, et al., 2000). The thalamic connection (lower loop on Figure 4-2 or low road on Figure 4-3) provides rapid and direct input concerning auditory signals, while cortical areas (higher loop on Figure 4-2 or high road on Figure 4-3) provide auditory information indirectly and more slowly (Iversen, Kupfermann, et al., 2000; P. J. Jastreboff, 2000; LeDoux, 1998). The direct signals from the thalamus are especially important to respond rapidly to situations of immediate danger. Stimulation of these auditory pathways from the thalamus and cortex results in long-term alterations of synaptic efficacy in the basolateral complex. These neural changes associated with learning are referred to as long-term potentiation (Chapman & Chattarji, 2000).

When a neutral sound is paired repeatedly with an offensively loud sound (unconditioned stimulus), the neutral sound (conditioned stimulus) will elicit by itself the same emotional reactions (conditioned response) caused by the noxious stimulus (Iversen, Kupfermann, et al., 2000). Studies have shown that subjects can be trained in this way to show symptoms of anxiety—perspiration and dry mouth—in response to a previously neutral sound. If the same training is performed on subjects with damage to the amygdala, they do not learn to react to the neutral sound, in spite of their conscious awareness that the neutral sound was paired with the loud sound. It now seems possible that storage of emotional memories involves not only the amygdala, but also the cingulate and parahippocampal cortices, which are connected to the amygdala.

Extinction

Pavlov (1927) was the first to use the term extinction. Extinction is the gradual inability of a CS to elicit a CR due to repeated presentation of the CS in the absence of a UCS with which the CS was originally paired (Falls, 1998). In essence, the CR stops occurring as a consequence of nonreinforcement. Pavlov (1927) also showed that an extinguished CR can recover to its original level ("spontaneous recovery") under certain circumstances (Falls, 1998).

Konorski (1948) updated Pavlov's concepts about extinction to be more consistent with advances in neurophysiology and provided a more detailed explanation of putative mechanisms of extinction (Falls, 1998). Konorski described classical conditioning with respect to neural centers that were activated by different stimuli. He surmised that pairing a CS with a UCS involves the progressive strengthening of excitatory connections between the corresponding neural centers. Once paired, activation of the CS center alone would, via the excitatory connections, produce activation of the UCS center, eliciting the CR. If, after pairing, the CS was presented repeatedly without the UCS, inhibitory connections would develop between the CS and UCS centers. With continued nonreinforcement, the inhibitory connections would strengthen to the point of becoming dominant over the excitatory connections—resulting in extinction of the CR. Konorski believed that spontaneous recovery was possible (as did Pavlov), which he explained was due to the excitatory associations between neural centers remaining intact during the process of establishing inhibitory connections. Konorski also believed, however, that continued nonreinforcement of a CS would eventually strengthen the inhibitory connections to the point that spontaneous recovery could not occur.

Instrumental Conditioning

With classical conditioning, an association is learned between two stimuli (Kandel et al., 2000). With instrumental conditioning, an association is learned between a behavior and a consequence. Also called operant conditioning or trial-and-error learning, instrumental conditioning is thought to govern the majority of human voluntary behavior. People and animals tend to repeat behaviors that are rewarded, and not repeat behaviors that have negative consequences. Although this method of learning appears to be different than classical conditioning, it is thought that the two forms of learning involve similar neural mechanisms.

Although the name B. F. Skinner is most often associated with instrumental conditioning, J. Konorski was the first to describe two types of conditioned reflexes—the second type being instrumental conditioning (Konorski, 1948; Konorski & Miller, 1937). Konorski's "type II conditioned reflex" contrasted with Pavlov's conditioned response (CR), which was a "type I conditioned reflex." There is thus a general dichotomization of behavior as either "operant" or "respondent" (Allan, 1998). This dichotomous approach may be due to the realization that the environment can interact with behavior in only two ways. (a) With operant behavior, there is a behavioral response followed by a reinforcer. In this case, a behavior is followed reliably by changes in the environment that feed back to determine the future probability of the behavior. (b) Respondent behavior involves a stimulus that is followed by a reinforcer. Respondent behavior is based on the ability of an unconditioned stimulus (US) to elicit a behavior without the need for any prior training. The response reliably follows the US, and does not generally occur in the absence of the US. While these two different types of behavior can be manipulated in the laboratory, in real life the shaping and maintenance of behavior are a complex mix of operant and respondent contingencies.

Habituation

The concept of habituation has been a part of the learning and conditioning literature for many years, and refers generally to a decrease in responsiveness as a result of repeated stimulation (Domjan & Burkhard, 1986; Konorski, 1948). More specifically, habituation is "a decrease in a behavioral reflex response to a repeated, non-noxious stimulus" (Kupfermann, 1985). The stimulus can be auditory, visual, or tactile. A novel, unexpected stimulus will initially elicit a startle (orienting) response, which can be observed as a sudden reaction involving a "jump" of the body immediately following the stimulus. Elicitation of the startle reflex is part of a behavioral auditory assessment for infants (Hodgson, 1994b). Examiners are cautioned, however, that the startle response tends to disappear rapidly when the stimulus is presented repeatedly. Thus, infants learn very quickly that the relatively intense tone has no informative or predictive value, and the response to the tone becomes habituated.

A key feature of habituation is its stimulus specificity, i.e., the reduction in responding is to some degree specific to the particular stimulus (Thompson & Donegan, 1987). If certain features of the stimulus are altered, then the habituated response will recover to some extent. In addition, the response decrement with repeated stimulation is greatest when the stimulus is weak, and reduced when the stimulus is intense.

Habituation is nonassociative learning and the simplest type of implicit learning (Kandel, 2000b). The effect has been studied extensively in animals, especially in the marine sea slug aplysia due to its extremely simple nervous system. Aplysia has a gill (respiratory organ) and a siphon that expels seawater and waste. Touching the siphon for the first time elicits the defensive gill-withdrawal reflex. With repeated stimulation, however, the reflex becomes progressively smaller, due to a reduction in synaptic effectiveness in the neural pathways mediating the reflex. The reduced synaptic effectiveness is the result of a chain of neural events leading to a decrease in transmitter release into the synapses throughout the reflex circuit. Thus, memory in such a case is not located at a single specialized site, but rather is distributed and stored throughout the circuit. This same general mechanism explains habituation in other animals, as well as habituation to the startle response in humans.

Habituation has been characterized as a simple type of learning, which is very similar to extinction of conditioned responses (Domjan & Burkhard, 1986; Thompson, 1967). Both types of learning involve repeated presentation of an unreinforced stimulus. The critical difference is that only extinction involves prior conditioning. Konorski (1948, p. 145) wrote:

> . . . the mechanism of extinction of the orientation reflex has to be thought of as analogous to that of extinction of the conditioned reflex. In other words, we assume that the gradual disappearance of the orientation reflex with the repetition of the corresponding stimulus is due to the formation of inhibitory connections between certain intervening centers in just the same way as they are formed in the extinction of the conditioned reflex. This would explain the striking similarity of the properties of these two processes. . . .

Konorski (1967, p. 99) later wrote:

> When a stimulus is repeatedly presented without being followed by any arousal-producing consequences, these effects are gradually attenuated and some of them may be eventually totally abolished. This phenomenon, originally denoted by Pavlov as "extinction of orientation reaction," is now usually called "habituation."

Thus, the terms *habituation*, *extinction of orienting reflex*, and *extinction of conditioned reflexes* (as well as the different versions of these terms) generally refer to the same phenomenon of a reduction in responding as a result of nonreinforcement. A further distinction has been made between "passive" and "active" extinction (Daw, Kakade, & Dayan, 2002). J. Konorski routinely made this distinction in his lectures, which is the source of the term *passive extinction of conditioned reflexes* that is equated with habituation. These terms are used interchangeably with respect to TRT.

Sensitization

Repeated stimulation with a harmless stimulus causes habituation. If a *harmful* stimulus is presented, however, the animal learns to react more vigorously to defend itself against the stimulus (Kandel, 2000b). Repeated presentation of the harmful stimulus enhances the reflexive reactions, and this enhancement is known as sensitization. Sensitization can also be caused by novel or appetitive stimuli (Thompson & Donegan, 1987).

Sensitization and habituation are the two major forms of nonassociative learning, but the cellular mechanisms that produce synaptic change in sensitization are different, and more complex, than those involved in habituation (Kandel, 2000b). With habituation, only synapses that are part of the reflex pathway are modified. With sensitization, additional neurons (modulatory interneurons) are activated to enhance synaptic strength. This mechanism for sensitization also results in a generalized state of readiness or arousal such that any stimulus, even a harmless stimulus, would cause a more vigorous response than normal. Such a nonspecific state of sensitization would describe a person who is "jumpy" and overreacts to a variety of stimuli.

HOW TINNITUS RELATES TO DIFFERENT FORMS OF LEARNING

Tinnitus becomes a clinical problem when the patient "learns" to connect it with a negative emotional response. The stress of tinnitus results from a perceived sound or auditory neural signal that by itself is harmless. The remainder of this chapter provides a theoretical discussion of how different types of learning might be involved in tinnitus becoming a clinically significant condition.

Tinnitus and Classical Conditioning

With respect to classical conditioning, tinnitus can be considered a neutral stimulus having the potential to acquire negative meaning via association with another stimulus. Using conditioning terminology, the tinnitus can become a conditioned stimulus (CS) when it is paired with an unconditioned stimulus (UCS) (see Table 6–1). The UCS has the innate quality of eliciting an unconditioned response (UCR). After pairing of the stimuli, the tinnitus can elicit the same response, which is now a conditioned response (CR). The circumstances under which a tinnitus signal acquires meaning are, of course, far more complex than this oversimplified description might imply. It is likely that almost all human responses are the result of a combination of classical and instrumental conditioning (Allan, 1998).

The tinnitus percept can be thought of as an auditory stimulus that may consist of one or multiple sounds, and may be constant, fluctuant, or intermittent. The sound may be perceived as weak or intense, and it can be similar in timbre (spectral characteristics) to external sounds. Any of these variable characteristics of tinnitus can influence how much attention is given to the signal, regardless of whether the tinnitus is associated with another stimulus. For example, intense tinnitus would be more salient than weak tinnitus, and tinnitus that sounds "scratchy" might be more attention-getting than tonal tinnitus. These aspects of the tinnitus sound and how they can independently affect tinnitus distress will be discussed further in the section Tinnitus and Sensitization below. For classical conditioning, the specifics of the sensory stimulus are secondary because any sound can be conditioned to evoke a specific reflexive emotional reaction.

For tinnitus to become a problem via classical conditioning, the tinnitus-related neural signal must acquire the meaning of another stimulus (UCS) that evokes negative emotions (UCR). This transfer of meaning results in a conditioned reflex (CR). If an association is made at the conscious level, then conscious attention directed to the tinnitus would cause a reaction as if the tinnitus was another stimulus. Thus, when attending consciously to the tinnitus (CS), the person reacts as if experiencing the associated emotion-provoking events (which describes the conditioned emotional response). For example, a soldier might have acquired tinnitus during combat and emotional responses are evoked whenever the aversive experience is recalled from memory. If an association has been established between the tinnitus and the combat experience, conscious awareness of the tinnitus might evoke the same emotional reactions as remembering the combat experience.

On the other hand, a person's tinnitus might be associated with a pleasurable (*appetitive*) event. A musician, for example, might be accustomed to returning home after a concert or rehearsal to a "ringing" or "hissing" sound in the ears that is obviously the result of the loud music. The musical activity is a pleasurable experience, however, so the persistent tinnitus does not trigger negative associations. As a result, when directing attention to the tinnitus, the musician might react as if recalling the musical experience—either with pleasant thoughts or with essentially no affect.

It is relevant to note that two studies support the notion that physical parameters of sound are not the only factors that influence the damaging effects of noise on the auditory system. Lindgren and Axelsson (1983) exposed subjects to music and noise that was acoustically matched to the music (equal level-, frequency-, and time-distribution characteristics). Sixty percent of the subjects experienced less temporary threshold shift (TTS) in response to the music than to the noise. (There were no differences in TTS for the remaining subjects.) Swanson, Dengerink, Kondrick, and Miller (1987) used two groups of subjects—those who liked and those who disliked pop/rock music. Both groups were exposed to music and to noise. Those who liked music experienced less TTS than those who disliked music. These studies provide evidence that cochlear damage in response to noise can be influenced by psychological factors. It is therefore conceivable that loud sound that is perceived with a positive attitude may have mitigating effects on the onset and intensity of tinnitus.

Nonconscious Learning

It needs to be emphasized that these kinds of emotional reactions can occur nonconsciously (i.e., without directing any conscious attention to the tinnitus). Conditioning can occur without the perception of a stimulus, as shown in the substantial literature on nonconscious learning and conditioning (e.g., LeDoux, 1998; Lewicki, Hill, & Czyzewska, 1992; Reber, 1989). Mineka and Hamida (1998, p. 428) have aptly described this phenomenon:

> Sometimes an individual does not recall any experience of acquisition (either a direct or an observational conditioning experience). It is not uncommon, for example, for an individual to not have a clear recollection of when certain symptoms began or what triggered their onset (e.g., Lazarus, 1971). Similarly, it is not uncommon to find that individuals may volunteer an answer to the question of what caused their fear but feel uncertain about their answer's validity. It may seem surprising that if learning is indeed involved, as we usually believe it is, the process or circumstances of acquisition would not have gone unnoticed or have been forgotten. However, this does seem to happen.

Although views about nonconscious learning are not consensual among researchers, certain characteristics distinguish the phenomenon from conscious learning (Mineka & Hamida, 1998). Cognitive psychology describes nonconscious learning as occurring automatically and without intention. Nonconscious learning is faster than conscious learning, involves the learning of much more complex information, and is not subject to voluntary control. Nonconscious learning also is difficult to influence by conscious thought or intention. The same principles apply to nonconscious extinction of conditioned reflexes.

Many tinnitus patients report that their tinnitus onset was not related to any known event (Meikle & Griest, 1989). Such cases of idiopathic tinnitus can cause a variety of concerns as the individual imagines what might be causing the tinnitus. These concerns can turn into worry and fear about the medical and/or psychiatric implications of the tinnitus. The person then becomes conditioned to react emotionally (conditioned response) whenever attention is given to the tinnitus because of the association of the tinnitus perception (conditioned stimulus) with thoughts of serious health consequences (unconditioned stimulus). The heightened perception of tinnitus and associated negative reactions comprise a positive feedback loop (the "vicious circle") that can result in a clinically significant tinnitus condition (J. A. Henry, Schechter, et al., 2002; P. J. Jastreboff et al., 1996; P. J. Jastreboff & Hazell, 1998).

Tinnitus and Instrumental Conditioning

People often learn behaviors that reduce the negative consequences of their tinnitus. Many patients report the discovery of certain sounds that provide a sense of relief from their tinnitus. Based on the principles of instrumental conditioning, these patients tend to perform behaviors that facilitate exposure to the palliative sounds. For example, they might discover that leaving a fan on in the bedroom facilitates sleep, or that maintaining background music makes it easier to concentrate on office work. Other patients report a great variety of techniques that they have found helpful for their tinnitus, especially their involvement in tasks that require focused attention (which directs their attention away from their tinnitus). Discovering these kinds of solutions involves trial-and-error learning, and many patients go to great lengths to identify sources of relief.

Tinnitus and Sensitization

Tinnitus can cause an emotional reaction independent of any other stimulus or event. Thus, nonassociative learning can occur to the tinnitus signal alone. If a person's tinnitus is not associated with any other stimulus, and the person reacts emotionally when directing attention to the tinnitus, then sensitization to the tinnitus has occurred.

It was mentioned above (in Tinnitus and Classical Conditioning) that the tinnitus percept can differ in a great number of ways—loudness (intensity), pitch, spectral characteristics (timbre), degree of constancy, similarity with other sounds, etc. Each of these perceptual attributes of tinnitus represents a factor that can contribute to the perceived prominence of the tinnitus, and therefore to the annoyance caused by the tinnitus. This effect is similar to the common observation that different environmental sounds cause different emotional states. People tend to listen to sounds that are pleasurable, and to avoid sounds that are aversive. Sounds vary in how they affect different individuals, as indicated by the diverse listening options on the radio, or by the different types of sounds that different people find annoying. In general, certain sounds are found to evoke pleasure, or to at least be innocuous (e.g., music, moving water, nature sounds), while other sounds are perceived as aversive (e.g., fingernails scratching a blackboard, buzzers, car rattles). The sound of clinically significant tinnitus is probably never reported by patients to be a pleasurable sound, and almost all patients state that it is annoying to some degree. Annoyance that is caused solely by the aversiveness or intrusiveness of the tinnitus sound is the result of sensitization. On the other hand, some people who simply "experience" tinnitus describe positive aspects of the sound (e.g., the sound of crickets or cicadas during a peaceful summer evening).

Sensitization to tinnitus can cause a person to become progressively more anxious. However, due to the generalized nature of sensitization (Thompson & Donegan, 1987), other factors might contribute to the sensitized state. For example, if the person is anxious for other reasons, this could enhance the reaction to the tinnitus. For a given individual with tinnitus, these kinds of interplays cannot be completely differentiated. An awareness of these various factors can help to identify the reasons why tinnitus is so bothersome for a particular patient, which can assist in focusing treatment most effectively.

Tinnitus and Habituation

Habituation is a key learning concept for TRT. The main goal of treatment is for patients to achieve a high degree of habituation to their tinnitus. It is estimated that 80% of individuals who experience chronic tinnitus habituate to their tinnitus naturally. The remaining 20% are typically considered candidates for clinical intervention aimed at promoting habituation of tinnitus reaction and perception (A. Davis & Refaie, 2000; P. J. Jastreboff & Hazell, 1998). These latter individuals spend a large percentage of their waking hours perceiving and reacting to their tinnitus.

Effectiveness of therapy is indicated in part by a significant reduction in patient reports of the percentage of their waking hours that they are aware of, and annoyed by, their tinnitus (as determined by Questions 7 and 8, respectively, from the TRT Follow-up Interview, Appendix B). The ultimate goal of TRT is for these ratings to drop to 0% (or at least very close to 0%). Such improvement would normally be corroborated by a report that quality of life has improved significantly as well as by reduced scores on tinnitus and mood rating scales.

Considering the model of habituation with respect to aplysia (discussed above in the section Habituation), the organism reacted vigorously when a tactile stimulus was first delivered to its siphon (Kandel, 2000b). The repeated contact was eventually perceived as harmless and thus resulted in progressively smaller reactions. It might seem that such a model would not be relevant to tinnitus, which typically has a gradual onset and is experienced as a constant stimulus. The concept of habituation, however, extends to all kinds of situations involving exposure to various stimuli (including tinnitus).

Directed attention, and its neural mechanisms, was discussed in Chapter 3. People are exposed to millions of sensory impulses at any given instant, and the CNS must sort and filter all of those impulses in real time so as to route only the most relevant information to cortical areas for conscious attention. A pair of glasses resting on the nose is an example of being exposed to a constant (tactile) stimulus without maintaining conscious awareness of its presence. This filtering and blocking mechanism enables people to ignore stimuli that are not relevant to the task at hand, while directing attention only to meaningful stimuli. Thus, the CNS processes all incoming stimuli subconsciously to facilitate organized, focused, and effective behavior. Tinnitus is just one of many signals that must be processed by the CNS. The neural mechanisms that are responsible for processing auditory signals cannot distinguish between normal auditory signals and tinnitus. Just as most auditory signals are normally habituated, tinnitus also can be habituated.

Recall (from the section Habituation) that habituation is stimulus specific (Thompson & Donegan, 1987). Thus, altering certain features of the stimulus can cause recovery of the habituated response (dishabituation). With regard to tinnitus, this might imply that tinnitus that undergoes changes in spectral characteristics (timbre) might be more difficult to habituate. Recall also that the terms *habituation*, *extinction of orienting reflex*, and *extinction of conditioned reflexes* refer essentially to the same phenomenon. In this regard, Konorski (1948) theorized that presentation of the conditioned stimulus (CS) is required for extinction (Falls, 1998). It is thus important that any learning (retraining) that takes place during TRT is to the "usual" (normally experienced) tinnitus percept; i.e., if the spectral characteristics of the tinnitus percept are altered, then learning (habituation) will not take place to the usual tinnitus. This is the rationale for ensuring that sound therapy always uses sound that is at or below the *mixing point* (as explained in Chapter 13). In the extreme situation, when the tinnitus signal cannot be detected (i.e., when it is completely suppressed or "masked"), by definition habituation to the signal cannot occur. This point is supported by the clinical observation of 20 patients who used masking for about 15 years without experiencing any reduction in tinnitus perception or annoyance (P. J. Jastreboff & Hazell, 2004). These patients were switched to a TRT protocol, received proper counseling, and were instructed to use ear-level sound at or below the mixing point. Each of these patients experienced full habituation to their tinnitus within a short period of initiating treatment with TRT.

SUMMARY AND DISCUSSION

Based on the discussion thus far, some basic premises can be made: (a) Tinnitus is a stimulus capable of evoking a learned response. (b) Tinnitus may evoke a learned response independent of any other stimulus (nonassociative learning), and/or it may become paired with another stimulus (resulting in a conditioned response). (c) Tinnitus can be considered an aversive stimulus by the person experiencing it, or it can be perceived as benign or innocuous. If the tinnitus is perceived as aversive, its aversiveness is a matter of degree (e.g., "mildly," "moderately," or "severely" aversive). Benign tinnitus would have no innate aversive qualities. (d) Although tinnitus is often perceived as fluctuating or intermittent, it is considered a constant sound by most patients (Meikle, Creedon, & Griest, 2004).

People who experience tinnitus generally became aware of its presence as a continuous internal sound at some specific point in time, regardless of whether the tinnitus was incurred gradually or more suddenly. At the time of this awareness, the tinnitus percept becomes a unique and identifiable stimulus capable of causing a variety of consequences that vary based on many factors. Because of the novelty and inescapability of new-onset tinnitus, the stimulus is likely to capture the person's attention during the initial period of awareness (due at least partly to the orienting reflex). Initial reactions can involve worry, anxiety, and fear, and these reactions can range from slight to catastrophic (McCombe et al., 2001). Over time, these initial reactions may increase or decrease. It was noted above (in the section Habituation) that habituation tends to occur most rapidly in response to a weak stimulus, but more slowly in response to an intense stimulus (Thompson & Donegan, 1987). Therefore, a decrease in the strength of the tinnitus signal by sound therapy is used to facilitate the process of habituation.

Increasing Reactions to Tinnitus

If a person's orienting reactions to the tinnitus onset increase over time, then either sensitization, classical conditioning, or a combination of the two will have occurred. Sensitization alone would imply that tinnitus is an aversive stimulus such as pain, loud noise, bitter taste, heat, or cold (Wilson, 2006). The nonassociative learning implicit with sensitization is due to the perceived aversiveness of the stimulus, which alone can be sufficient to cause sustained reactions. An example of an aversive auditory stimulus is a dripping water faucet. The sound may be barely audible, but it can prevent a person from falling asleep due to its incessant repetition. A much louder sound may be present while attempting to fall asleep, such as a fan, tabletop sound generator, or even traffic noise, but these kinds of sounds are easily habituated and do not interfere with sleep (they can actually aid sleep). There are always exceptions to these generalities—different people have different perceptions about what kinds of sounds are aversive.

Classical conditioning is involved if the tinnitus becomes associated, or linked, with another stimulus. Tinnitus that is a consequence of a traumatic experience such as a car accident or a military combat situation can become mentally and emotionally linked with the memories of the trauma. Directing attention to the tinnitus can trigger these negative memories resulting in emotional reactions as if reacting to the trauma experience itself. This associative learned response can be active at nonconscious levels (as explained in detail in Chapter 4, and in the section Nonconscious Learning above), which would cause the tinnitus signal to function as a continuous trigger to the amygdala where emotional memories are stored. The amygdala in turn activates the hypothalamus and sympathetic division of the autonomic nervous system, which can result in a chronic state of stress.

Decreasing Reactions to Tinnitus

Many people who initially experience tinnitus may react at first, but their reactions decrease over time (Dobie, 2004b; Hallam, Rachman, & Hinchcliffe, 1984). This decay in reactivity can be due to habituation of reaction, which is also referred to as passive extinction of conditioned reflexes (see section Habituation above). The crucial factor to successfully induce and sustain habituation of reaction is to reclassify the tinnitus to the category of a neutral stimulus, so the perception of tinnitus carries no inherent meaning (P. J. Jastreboff & Hazell, 2004). For habituation to occur, the perceived aversiveness of the tinnitus must not be so great as to cause a sustained reaction (i.e., sensitization). For example, if a fan runs continuously in the background, it is normally habituated. If a rattling sound develops while the fan is running, however, the noise of the fan takes on an aversive quality. Because of its aversiveness, the rattling fan cannot be ignored, and action must be taken to correct the annoying sound. Once corrected, the fan again becomes an innocuous sound that can be easily habituated.

When an association develops between the tinnitus percept and the memory of an event, the association is usually negative, but can also be positive (or neutral). The musician hearing tinnitus after performing in a concert is an example of a positive/neutral association (although all musicians do not necessarily react in this manner). When a negative association develops, any decrease in reactions requires extinction of conditioned reflexes. Conditioned responses are extinguished when the value of the conditioned stimulus (CS) is reduced by failure to present the unconditioned stimulus (UCS). In the case of tinnitus (the CS), its significance is reduced when there is a reduction in the emotional memories (the UCS) that are associated with the tinnitus.

CONCLUSION

People who experience tinnitus live their lives in the presence of an intrusive and inescapable auditory stimulus. Many factors interact to determine whether the stimulus will cause emotional reactions and stress in a given individual. Any form of therapy should attempt to minimize these reactions. TRT attempts to accomplish this goal through specific clinical protocols of education and sound therapy (P. J. Jastreboff & Hazell, 2004). The education focuses on the neurophysiological model in the attempt to "devalue" the phantom auditory stimulus. With sound therapy a constant background of nonannoying sound is maintained for the purpose of reducing the strength and detectability of the stimulus.

The educational counseling that is described for TRT in Chapter 13 uses certain learning terminology that has been defined in the present chapter. Mostly, the terms *passive extinction of conditioned reflexes* and *habituation* are used interchangeably to describe the overall process of reducing emotional and autonomic reactions to tinnitus through the modification of connections and/or alteration of neural activity between the auditory nervous system and the limbic and autonomic nervous systems. TRT counseling is designed to explain to the patient, from a neurophysiological perspective, how the tinnitus neural signal causes significant emotional and autonomic reactions, and how the brain can be retrained through counseling and appropriate acoustic stimulation to process the signal differently with the aim of mitigating the negative reactions (P. J. Jastreboff & Hazell, 2004).

PART 2

Clinical Guidelines for Assessment

Clinical implementation of TRT involves three basic components: assessment of the patient to determine treatment needs, structured educational counseling, and a prescribed program of sound therapy. The assessment protocol is described in Part 2 and the treatment protocols are described in Part 3.

7

Referral Guidelines

The issue of referring tinnitus patients is largely a matter of professional perspective—there is no consensus due to the multiple and diverse health care fields that are involved in managing tinnitus patients. These fields include otolaryngology, otology, otoneurology, neurotology, psychiatry, audiology, psychology, and others (including numerous alternative and complementary specialties). Depending on the particular field, any referral recommendations would tend to reflect the field's specific management approach. Even within each field there are no consensual guidelines. This lack of consensus of course extends beyond just referral issues—tinnitus management in general does not adhere to any standard of practice (Dobie, 2004a). The referral guidelines that are recommended here should adequately address the needs of most tinnitus patients.

The health care disciplines that are most commonly involved in tinnitus management are otolaryngology/otology, psychology, and audiology. From the otolaryngological/otological perspective, it has been argued that all tinnitus patients should receive a complete head and neck examination (Perry & Gantz, 2000). Tinnitus professionals in the field of psychology argue that tinnitus distress is a psychological problem that would indicate the need for psychological management (J. L. Henry & Wilson, 2001). The American Speech-Language-Hearing Association includes tinnitus in its scope of practice for audiologists (ASHA, 2004), and it has been argued that audiologists are the best qualified to provide the majority of tinnitus clinical services (J. A. Henry, 2004; J. A. Henry, Zaugg, & Schechter, 2005).

Clearly, there are many perspectives concerning the question of which health care specialty should serve as primary providers for tinnitus patients. A true multidisciplinary approach would require tinnitus patients to undergo appropriate medical, psychological, and audiological evaluations. Treatment would involve some combination of approaches from these different disciplines. This is certainly the ideal, and should be the standard of practice whenever possible. However, maintaining such a standard would normally require patients to attend separate appointments in multiple clinics, which is not realistic for patients who often report their tinnitus to be nothing more than a nuisance. Even for patients with more severe tinnitus, receiving multidisciplinary care would require the various disciplines to work together as a multidisciplinary team, which is seldom the case.

At a minimum, tinnitus patients should receive a complete hearing assessment and be screened properly for common comorbid mental health conditions (J. A. Henry, Zaugg, et al., 2005). The examiner should be fully qualified to perform all of the necessary testing. Normally, an audiologist is in the position of performing this testing independently, or in conjunction with an associated physician or mental health professional. An essential component of the tinnitus intake assessment is determining if the patient requires referral for a medical and/or a psychological evaluation.

Patients should always be referred for evaluation by an otologist or otolaryngologist whenever symptoms suggest the presence of a vestibular schwannoma (also known as acoustic neuroma or acoustic neurinoma) or Ménière's disease. Audiologists are trained in the identification of these symptoms. Vestibular schwannomas are unilateral 95% of the time (National Institutes of Health Consensus [NIH], 1994). The most common symptom of vestibular schwannoma is unilateral, progressive hearing loss (occasionally the hearing loss can be sudden). The second most common symptom of vestibular schwannoma is unilateral tinnitus, which patients usually describe as a high-pitched ringing sound. Classic symptoms of Ménière's disease include low-pitched tinnitus, low-frequency sensorineural hearing loss, vertigo, and aural fullness. All of these Ménière's symptoms tend to be of a fluctuating nature.

It is important to distinguish between sensorineural tinnitus and *somatosounds*. Sensorineural tinnitus (or just *tinnitus*) has a neurophysiological origin, whereas somatosounds can be generated from vascular, muscular, or respiratory sources (Hazell, 1995). Somatosounds can also be produced by the temporomandibular joint (Chole & Parker, 1992). Rarely, somatosounds are "objective," i.e., they can occasionally be heard by the examiner (Møller, 2003). Because somatosounds by definition have an acoustic source, all somatosounds theoretically should be physically detectable if the proper equipment and techniques were available. The most common somatosound is *pulsatile tinnitus*, i.e., tinnitus that is synchronous with the heart beat (Lockwood et al., 2004; Sismanis, 1998; Wackym & Friedland, 2004). Based on clinical observations, it can be theorized that fluctuations in tinnitus loudness may be synchronized with the heartbeat even when there is no somatosound, as heartbeat related changes in the pressure of cerebrospinal fluid, and therefore perilymph, may affect functioning of the cochlea. Since somatosounds are potentially correctable surgically, a complete head and neck examination should be conducted whenever they are suspected (Perry & Gantz, 2000; Wackym & Friedland, 2004). TRT is effective in treating somatosounds as well as tinnitus.

Although a thorough medical examination (otoneurology and/or neurotology; otolaryngology and/or neurology) is always in the patient's best interest, it is often done only to rule out medically correctable causes of tinnitus. The most common form of tinnitus is neurophysiological tinnitus that is consistent with sensorineural hearing loss and a history of noise exposure. These patients often report tinnitus that has been fairly stable for years. Tinnitus described in this way is not correctable surgically, nor is it life-threatening.

MENTAL HEALTH CONCERNS

Anxiety and Depression

Tinnitus patients are disproportionately affected by depression and anxiety (Dobie, 2004b). When either of these conditions coexists with tinnitus, it is essential that the patient receives proper treatment from a mental health provider. Questionnaires are available to determine if a mental health referral would be appropriate. For depression, the Beck Depression Inventory (BDI) is considered a standard assessment tool (Beck, Ward, Mendelson, Mock, & Erbaugh, 1961). The BDI can be completed in about 5 minutes. There are also screening versions of the BDI, including a 13-item version (Dobie & Sullivan, 1998). The most recent BDI is the BDI-II, which can be ordered online at http://www.harcourtassessment.com. For anxiety, the Spielberger State-Trait Anxiety Inventory is often used, which requires approximately 10 minutes for the patient to self-administer (Spielberger, 1983). It is available for purchase from http://www.mindgarden.com/products/staisad.htm. There is also a six-item short form of the state scale of the Spielberger State-Trait Anxiety Inventory, but it has not been validated. These depression and anxiety questionnaires can be administered by non-mental health clinicians, provided there is no diagnostic interpretation of the test scores (J. A. Henry, Zaugg, et al., 2005). The mood-rating scales suggested here are just some of the many good scales that are available.

Post-Traumatic Stress Disorder

A psychological disorder that often goes unrecognized is post-traumatic stress disorder (PTSD). Common symptoms of PTSD are nightmares, flashbacks, exaggerated startle responses, and excessive anxiety or fear. These symptoms can follow the experience of a traumatic event and can be present in any patient. For United States citizens, it has been estimated that about 61% of men and 51% of women have experienced at least one traumatic event, and that 5% of men and 10% of women experience PTSD at some time in their lives (Department of Veterans Affairs, 2005). Untreated PTSD can impair any efforts to treat tinnitus. If the clinician suspects PTSD, then the Primary Care PTSD screening tool (PC-PTSD) is available to assist in determining need for referral (Department of Veterans Affairs, 2005).

Insomnia

Tinnitus patients report sleep disturbance more than any other tinnitus-related problem (Axelsson & Ringdahl, 1989; Jakes, Hallam, Chambers, & Hinchcliffe, 1985; Meikle et al., 2004; Tyler & Baker, 1983). Patients who report sleep disturbance also tend to be those with the most problematic tinnitus (Erlandsson, Hallberg, & Axelsson, 1992; Folmer & Griest, 2000; Meikle, Vernon, & Johnson, 1984; Scott, Lindberg, Melin, & Lyttkens, 1990). For these patients, bedside augmentative sound (e.g., digital music player, tabletop sound generator, sound pillow, fan) is crucial and may be sufficient to mitigate the sleep problems. There are even some ear-level devices that are appropriate for wearing during sleep (e.g., some in-the-ear or micro behind-the-ear sound generators). If the sleep problem is severe, it may be appropriate to refer the patient to a sleep disorders clinic, or to an appropriate physician or mental health professional.

Medications

There are numerous reports of prescription drugs being used to manage tinnitus, which has inspired many research studies to evaluate the efficacy of different drugs for this purpose. R. A. Dobie reviewed these studies and concluded that no drug has been shown to provide consistent benefit for tinnitus (Dobie, 1999, 2004a; Robinson, Viirre, & Stein, 2004). Drug treatment, however, may be warranted when a patient has, for example, a high level of comorbid anxiety, depression, obsessive-compulsive disorder, psychosis (and other *significant* disorders of mood and thought), chronic pain, seizures, and/or sleep disorder. Patients suspected of having a psychological disorder should be referred to a mental health professional. Thus, drugs may be useful to treat a psychological disorder, but they are not generally recommended to treat tinnitus as an independent condition.

There are a few conditions for which medications may be helpful in reducing the tinnitus perception and/or potentially minimizing cochlear hair cell damage: (a) bilateral anacusis (complete deafness), (b) profound hearing loss (with or without hearing aids), (c) sudden sensorineural hearing loss from noise trauma, and (d) prolonged tinnitus exacerbations. There are cases of patients who have severe to profound hearing loss for whom hearing aids are insufficient in facilitating an adequate degree of sound therapy. In these cases, certain medications are potentially helpful.

8

Self-Report Questionnaires

Tinnitus is a subjective symptom, and its clinical assessment relies mainly on the use of questionnaires. Questionnaires can be both written and verbal and are useful and essential in the assessment process (J. A. Henry, Zaugg, et al., 2005). In this brief chapter we will discuss the use of written questionnaires that would be considered supplementary to the TRT Initial Interview. Detailed guidelines for administering the Initial Interview are provided in Chapter 10.

Numerous self-assessment questionnaires for tinnitus have been developed with the purpose of providing an index score that quantifies the severity of a patient's tinnitus condition. The reader is referred to an excellent review of tinnitus questionnaires by Newman and Sandridge (2004). There are at least a dozen published tinnitus questionnaires, but none has achieved universal acceptance (Dobie, 2002; Meikle & Griest, 2002; Tyler, 1993). At present, work is in progress among tinnitus specialists to draft a more unifying tinnitus rating scale that will serve as an effective outcome measure and hopefully become the standard instrument for assessing tinnitus severity and outcomes of treatment (Meikle et al., 2005; Meikle, Abrams, Newman, Sandridge, & J. A. Henry, 2005).

Every tinnitus patient should complete a tinnitus questionnaire. Of the many tinnitus questionnaires available, it is essential to select one that has been documented for validity and reliability (Newman & Sandridge, 2004). Numerous questionnaires meet these criteria, making it difficult to decide which one would be best for common use. We recommend the Tinnitus Handicap Inventory (THI) because of its thorough documentation and widespread acceptance (Newman, Jacobson, & Spitzer, 1996; Newman, Sandridge, & Jacobson, 1998). The THI contains 25 questions that can be answered *yes* (4 points), *no* (0 points), or *sometimes* (2 points), for a total possible index score of 100 points (with higher scores indicating greater perceived handicap). Patients can be categorized as having mild (18–36 points), moderate (38–56 points), or severe (58–100 points) tinnitus handicap (or no handicap if the index score is 16 or less). The THI has been documented for internal consistency reliability (Cronbach's $\alpha = .93$) and test-retest reliability ($r = .92$) (Newman et al., 1998). It has also been shown that a change in the total index score of at least 20 points indicates a statistically and clinically significant change in self-perceived tinnitus handicap at the 95% confidence level (Newman & Sandridge, 2004).

While the index score of self-perceived tinnitus handicap is essential in the assessment of tinnitus patients, it should not be relied upon totally to reveal the true severity of the condition. Index scores can over- or underestimate the impact of tinnitus on a patient's life (J. A. Henry, Dennis, & Schechter, 2005). While there are hundreds of questions that could be asked about the consequences of tinnitus, a tinnitus questionnaire is limited to relatively few questions. A questionnaire addresses the most common issues reported by "typical" tinnitus patients. Many patients, however, are atypical in how they are affected by tinnitus, and the questionnaire may not be relevant to their unique issues.

Another limitation of questionnaires is that they weight all questions equally in calculating the index score (J. A. Henry, Dennis, et al., 2005). A patient who has a single problem with tinnitus may not provide an accurate index score, especially if the single problem is severe. That is, tinnitus may affect only one aspect of a patient's life, but if that one aspect is severely affected, the index score might underestimate the true impact of the tinnitus on the patient's life. This limitation can be partly overcome by the use of subscales. For example, the THI was designed so that questions were grouped into categories that evaluated functional, emotional, and "catastrophic" effects of tinnitus. In this way, each subscale provides its own index score. In some cases a subscale index score will be more representative of the tinnitus severity than the overall index score.

Tinnitus questionnaires are further limited in that they cannot guide the decision-making process to determine the type and degree of treatment that would be most appropriate for an individual patient. Making these kinds of decisions requires conducting an in-depth interview with the patient. Structured interview forms have been developed for this purpose (J. A. Henry, M. M. Jastreboff, P. J. Jastreboff, Schechter, & Fausti, 2003; J. A. Henry, Zaugg, et al., 2005; M. M. Jastreboff & P. J. Jastreboff, 1999; Schechter & J. A. Henry, 2002). TRT of course uses the TRT Initial Interview, described in detail in Chapter 10 and shown in Appendix A. A modified version of the Initial Interview is also available to monitor effects of treatment (TRT Follow-Up Interview, described in Chapter 14 and shown in Appendix B).

In summary, administration of the written THI and the TRT Interviews is recommended at every major treatment appointment. Decisions regarding therapy should be determined primarily by the patient's responses to the TRT Interviews. The corresponding THI index score will generally corroborate the interview responses. Effectiveness of therapy can be further indicated by reductions in different scales that rate depression, anxiety, sleep quality, and quality of life (some of which are described in Chapter 7). Most of these scales are used with adults but there are also scales that are specific to children. Choosing the most revealing and practical scales to use in routine practice is an individual preference, but some scales have been proven to be more scientifically robust than others.

9

Patient Treatment Categories

The TRT assessment involves interviewing the patient using the TRT Initial Interview (Appendix A), conducting an audiological assessment, and performing psychoacoustic testing to quantify the perceptual characteristics of the patient's tinnitus. Administering the Initial Interview can require up to 1 hour, and the audiological and psychoacoustic testing can require up to 2 hours. It is therefore suggested that 3 hours be allotted for the assessment appointment.

The primary purpose of the assessment is to identify the patient's TRT category, which will determine the overall course of treatment most suitable for the patient. There are five basic categories, in addition to subcategories. Because each patient has unique needs, the categories should be used only as a general guide. Flexibility is required to adapt the treatment protocols to the patient's specific needs. When the assessment has been completed, the clinician and patient should discuss the test results and work together to achieve mutual agreement concerning the most appropriate course of action. Prior to making any commitment to undergo treatment, the patient must fully understand the objectives of treatment, the treatment schedule, requirements for using ear-level devices, costs, and any other details of the planned treatment.

The basic TRT patient categories include 0, 1, 2, 3, and 4 (P. J. Jastreboff, 1998; P. J. Jastreboff & Hazell, 2004) (Table 9-1). Assigning patients accurately to one of the categories relies primarily on the responses obtained during administration of the TRT Initial Interview. The audiometric data are also essential, but the Interview provides the means to clearly differentiate between the patient's perception of any difficulties relating to tinnitus, hearing loss, and decreased tolerance of sound. It can often be difficult for the patient to make a clear distinction between these three issues, and the Interview is structured to facilitate

TABLE 9–1. Criteria for Assigning TRT Patient Categories.

Patient Category	Criteria
0	✓ Tinnitus a minimal (or very recent) problem ✓ Hearing difficulties irrelevant
1	✓ Tinnitus a significant problem ✓ No significant problem with hearing loss
2	✓ Tinnitus a significant problem ✓ Hearing loss a significant problem
3	✓ Sound tolerance a significant problem ✓ Hearing difficulties irrelevant ✓ Tinnitus irrelevant
4	✓ Tinnitus and/or sound tolerance a significant problem ✓ Prolonged tinnitus and/or hyperacusis exacerbation caused by sound ✓ Hearing difficulties irrelevant

this process. Proper patient categorization relies on the accurate assessment of the relative impact of tinnitus, hearing loss, and decreased sound tolerance on the patient's life. Most importantly, this process is empowering to the patient by providing a clear understanding of exactly what problems need to be addressed.

CATEGORY 0

Category 0 defines patients whose problem with tinnitus is minimal or their tinnitus onset is very recent. These patients normally require only basic counseling, which should include a clear description of the need to maintain an enriched sound environment. Certain information may be purposefully omitted from the counseling if necessary to avoid overemphasis of tinnitus or presenting it as worse than it really is. These patients do not need to use ear-level sound generators, although the use of sound generators is certainly an option if so desired. Following their assessment, these patients should receive counseling that includes a description of the neurophysiological model (Chapter 13). The information gained by patients during the assessment, the post-assessment discussion, and the counseling is often sufficient to resolve most of their concerns. These patients should, however, return to the clinic 3–6 months later to ensure that any reported problems have been fully resolved. Category 0 patients should also be instructed to telephone the clinician if there is any exacerbation of symptoms. It is important to immediately address any concerns that could result in a worsening of the condition. In particular, if the patient has tinnitus of recent onset, the tinnitus condition needs to be monitored very carefully.

Category 0 patients may or may not have a problem with their hearing. If they do, they should be advised strongly to obtain hearing aids to improve their hearing. Patients with hearing loss and tinnitus often consider their tinnitus to be the root cause of their hearing difficulties (Coles, 1995; Dobie, 2004b; J. A. Henry, Zaugg, et al., 2005; Zaugg, Schechter, Fausti, & Henry, 2002). The tinnitus is a constantly perceptible symptom whereas the hearing loss is only noticed during certain situations. It is thus natural that some patients would make the assumption that the tinnitus is the cause of their hearing difficulties. The audiological assessment will identify any reduced hearing sensitivity, which is often discovered to be a high-frequency hearing loss that would create difficulties hearing in a background of noise. The patient should be counseled that any reported hearing difficulties are a result of the reduced hearing sensitivity. The use of hearing aids would alleviate this problem, and should provide the secondary benefit of reducing awareness of the tinnitus (J. A. Henry, Zaugg, et al., 2005; Searchfield, 2005).

CATEGORY 1

Category 1 patients require substantially more treatment than just basic counseling. These patients have tinnitus that is so problematic that an aggressive and proactive program of treatment is needed. Their tinnitus bothers them to such a degree that at least one major life activity is significantly affected (e.g., sleep, work, concentration), as normally determined by Question 12 from the TRT Initial Interview (Appendix A). Category 1 patients normally require at least 1 year of treatment that involves a protocol of repeated counseling and daily use of ear-level sound generators. Making a commitment to undergo this level of treatment requires an accurate assessment of the problem, which relies mainly on the information gained from conducting the Initial Interview. It is essential that both the patient and clinician are convinced that the treatment is necessary before undertaking Category 1 intervention.

CATEGORY 2

Category 2 patients also require an aggressive program of treatment for their tinnitus, but in addition they report significant hearing difficulties that affect quality of life. Results of audiological testing are helpful in making this determination, but the decision to use amplification should not be based on the test results alone. The critical factor in assigning a patient to Category 2 is that hearing loss has a significant impact on the patient's life, independent of the results of any hearing tests. It is especially important to ensure that the reported tinnitus problem is not really a hearing problem that is being blamed on the tinnitus. This can be adequately determined only through careful questioning using the Initial Interview.

Category 2 patients receive the same intervention as for Category 1 patients except that they wear either hearing aids or combination instruments. (Combination instruments incorporate both a hearing aid and a sound generator.) The primary purpose of the ear-level devices is to enrich the sound environment throughout each day, which is necessary to achieve long-term habituation of tinnitus. Improved hearing is considered a secondary objective for the use of these devices. In addition, the use of hearing aids plays a role by decreasing the "strain to hear" phenomenon (P. J. Jastreboff & Hazell, 2004). That is, straining to hear enhances the perception of tinnitus and hearing aids reduce this effect.

CATEGORY 3

Category 3 patients have a significant problem with decreased tolerance to sound. Specifically, they have the condition of hyperacusis. These patients are assigned to Category 3 regardless of whether they also have a significant problem with tinnitus. Treatment focuses on the hyperacusis for Category 3 patients. Once the hyperacusis condition is sufficiently resolved, the treatment then focuses on the tinnitus—assuming the tinnitus is a problem requiring treatment (which is usually the case). It is critical that there is a clear understanding of the definition of hyperacusis, which differs from misophonia and phonophobia. These terms are now defined as they apply to TRT.

Hyperacusis has been defined differently by different authors (P. J. Jastreboff & M. M. Jastreboff, 2004; Vernon, 2002). Vernon and Press (1998) defined it as "the collapse of loudness tolerance so that almost all sounds produce loudness discomfort" (p. 223). This definition would describe the stereotypical patient who cannot leave home without wearing earplugs and/or earmuffs due to an extreme problem tolerating environmental sounds. Such a patient would be very different from the up to 45% of patients that different clinics have reported to experience hyperacusis (Coles, 1996; Gold, Frederick, & Formby, 1999; Hazell, 1999; P. J. Jastreboff, 2000). Regardless of the precise definition, what matters is whether the patient has a significant problem with decreased sound tolerance. If so, the patient is diagnosed as hyperacusic, assigned to Category 3, and treated accordingly.

Hyperacusis is technically a physical condition of hypersensitivity of the auditory pathways, which is to be distinguished from misophonia. Misophonia describes decreased loudness tolerance involving the limbic and autonomic nervous systems, and is not a condition of the auditory nervous system (M. M. Jastreboff & P. J. Jastreboff, 2002). Whereas hyperacusis causes discomfort or pain in response to sound that reaches a certain level, misophonia is dislike of certain sounds due to those sounds' ability to cause negative emotional reactions. Misophonic reactions are learned responses; thus, one sound might be bothersome in some situations but not in others. Phonophobia refers to the fear of sound, which is a specific variation of misophonia when fear is the dominant emotion evoked by sound (P. J. Jastreboff & M. M. Jastreboff, 2000, 2003).

Normally, hyperacusis, misophonia, and phonophobia are all present to some extent when loudness tolerance is a significant problem. Severe hyperacusis naturally results in the development of misophonia (P. J. Jastreboff & M. M. Jastreboff, 2003). Mild hyperacusis may or may not involve misophonia. Misophonia also can be an isolated condition, developing independently as a result of negative experiences involving sound. The patient's psychological characteristics may play a role in the development of misophonia. The crucial point is that misophonia requires a treatment protocol different from that used for hyperacusis.

It is important not to confuse these related loudness tolerance conditions with loudness recruitment, which refers to abnormally rapid growth in the perception of loudness (Mencher, Gerber, & McCombe, 1997; Vernon, 1976, 2002). Recruitment is usually a symptom of cochlear or sensorineural hearing loss. Recruitment does not require treatment, but is a normal consequence of reduced hearing thresholds. The accelerated growth in loudness is caused by the reduced hearing thresholds, which result in a compressed dynamic range. The distinguishing features of loudness recruitment are reduced auditory sensitivity and normal loudness discomfort levels (LDLs).

The diagnosis of hyperacusis is made primarily on the basis of the patient's responses to the Sound Tolerance section of the TRT Initial Interview (Appendix A), which is usually corroborated by the finding of reduced LDLs. When a true condition of hyperacusis exists, LDLs at audiometric frequencies are observed to average less than 100 dB HL (P. J. Jastreboff, 2000). In a patient with "pure" misophonia, reduced LDLs might be present (e.g., when misophonic reactions exist to all sounds "louder than" a certain level), or alternatively might be normal because misophonic reactions may not include pure tones that are used to measure LDLs. If both hyperacusis and misophonia are present (as is always the case with severe hyperacusis), the average LDLs will be below 100 dB HL due to the hyperacusis component.

CATEGORY 4

Category 4 patients are relatively uncommon. They are, however, the patients who are most difficult to treat successfully (P. J. Jastreboff, 1998, 1999a). These patients experience tinnitus and/or hyperacusis that is made significantly worse after exposure to certain types of sounds. (Most Category 4 patients experience both tinnitus and hyperacusis.) More specifically, their problem is a prolonged exacerbation of tinnitus intensity, and/or of sensitivity to sound, that results from exposure to sound. The types of sounds that cause this effect would not be in the intensity range that would cause auditory damage. The defining feature of Category 4 patients is that their tinnitus/hyperacusis exacerbation lasts until at least the following day (after a night's sleep). Category 4 patients frequently have neurological problems induced by, for example, head injury, stroke, or Lyme disease.

The effect of tinnitus or hyperacusis exacerbation has been referred to as "kindling" or "winding-up" (P. J. Jastreboff, 1999a, 2000). The term *kindling* has been used to describe the inducement of epileptogenic responses in response to weak but repeated electrical stimulation to selected areas of the brain (Garnes & Pinel, 2001; Weiss, Li, Sitcoske-O'Shea, & Post, 2000). Stimulation of limbic structures in this manner was observed to cause a gradual increase in the extent and duration of the response, eventually inducing a generalized seizure (Westbrook, 2000). It has also been shown that audiogenic seizures can be evoked by exposing animals to loud sound using a similar approach (Feng & Faingold, 2002).

The term *winding-up* derives from the pain field. Tinnitus and pain have often been noted as being similar in many respects (Tonndorf, 1995). Winding-up refers to an increase in pain caused by prolonged exposure to a stimulus. Specifically, the stimulus initially does not cause pain, but low-level pain ensues with continued stimulation. Nociceptors are the receptors for painful stimuli, which are primarily free nerve endings embedded in peripheral tissues. When a painful stimulus is applied, both a fast, sharp pain and a slow, dull pain are experienced. The slow, dull pain is transmitted by unmyelinated C nerve fibers. Winding-up occurs when severe and persistent injury causes these C fibers to fire repetitively, which results in a gradual increase in the activity of central pain-mediating neurons (Basbaum & Jessell, 2000). The synaptic changes elicited by these central neurons occur over an extended period. This phenomenon is similar to long-term memory storage in the hippocampus (i.e., long-term potentiation) (Martinez & Derrick, 1996).

The TRT Initial Interview (Appendix A) contains questions that are designed specifically to reveal whether exposure to certain sounds results in prolonged exacerbation of tinnitus and/or hyperacusis. The responses to these questions are critical in determining if the patient should be placed in Category 4. The issue of prolonged exacerbation is addressed in Question 8 for tinnitus, and in Question 22 for hyperacusis. Because of the seriousness of the condition, and the difficulty treating it effectively, it is critically important to properly identify the condition to optimize the potential for a successful treatment outcome. The Initial Interview is particularly important as some misophonia patients may report the same perception of prolonged worsening.

10

TRT Initial Interview

Assessment of patients for treatment with TRT requires use of the TRT Initial Interview (Appendix A). As patients return for ongoing treatment, the TRT Follow-up Interview is used (Appendix B). The Follow-up Interview is a version of the Initial Interview that is modified to evaluate effects of treatment on the patient.

The original TRT interview forms were developed to facilitate the interview process with patients (M. M. Jastreboff & P. J. Jastreboff, 1999). These one-page forms are adequate for use by the experienced TRT clinician. The brevity of the forms, however, precludes asking the questions in a consistent manner by less experienced TRT providers. Consistency of form administration and scoring was critical for a controlled clinical trial that was conducted at the Portland (Oregon) VA Medical Center (J. A. Henry et al., 2006a,b). The forms were therefore expanded into fully scripted versions to provide this needed consistency (J. A. Henry et al., 2003). In addition, patient response options were modified and expanded to facilitate the acquisition of specific answers from a closed set of choices for each question. Restricting the response choices in this way provided data more readily amenable to statistical analysis. The scripted forms shown in Appendices A and B make it convenient for TRT clinicians to maintain consistency in the interview process and to enable direct comparison of data between clinics.

Conducting the TRT Initial Interview is the first step in the initial assessment appointment. Prior to meeting with the patient, however, there is first the need to review any written questionnaires and forms that the patient might have completed and provided to the clinic (see Chapter 8). The Tinnitus Handicap Inventory, and potentially other self-administered tinnitus questionnaires, should be reviewed to gain an overall perspective of the patient's tinnitus problem. Some clinics require that prospective patients complete special intake forms. These should also be reviewed prior to the initial appointment. Obtaining this information beforehand improves the efficiency of the assessment appointment.

ADDRESSING THE COMPLAINT THAT TINNITUS IMPAIRS HEARING

When administering the TRT Initial Interview, it is helpful to be aware that tinnitus can cause any or all of three fundamental problems in a person's life: (a) emotional reactions, (b) sleep disturbance, and (c) interference with concentration (Dobie, 2004b; J. A. Henry, Dennis, et al., 2005; Tyler, Noble, Preece, Dunn, & Witt, 2004). Although a multitude of complaints can be attributed to tinnitus, the complaints will fit generally into one or more of these three broad (and overlapping) categories. In addition, patients often claim that tinnitus interferes with their ability to hear. Attributing hearing loss to tinnitus can be a critical issue to address with patients. Some clarification of this issue is therefore necessary prior to describing the TRT Initial Interview.

It is the opinion of most tinnitus professionals that patients' claims of hearing problems caused by tinnitus are generally unwarranted, and are likely due to undiagnosed or unrecognized hearing loss (Coles, 1995; Dobie, 2004b; J. A. Henry, Dennis, et al., 2005; Zaugg et al., 2002). Hearing loss occurs gradually with aging, even when noise exposure is not a factor (Gordon-Salant, 2005; Pearson et al., 1995). The loss can be accelerated by noise exposure, ototoxicity, and otologic disease. This is especially common for noise, as, for example, over 30 million Americans are exposed to hazardous levels of noise on a regular basis (NIDCD, 2004). The relation between hearing loss and tinnitus is well documented (Axelsson & Barrenas, 1992; A. Davis & Refaie, 2000; Meikle, 1991a), and the majority of tinnitus patients experience hearing impairment to some degree (Axelsson & Ringdahl, 1989; A. Davis & Refaie, 2000; J. L. Henry & Wilson, 2001; Vernon, 1998). It is therefore not surprising that patients often confuse effects of hearing loss with effects of tinnitus.

The common scenario for a patient who attributes hearing problems to tinnitus is as follows. As presbycusis or noise-induced hearing loss develops, the person starts to notice difficulty understanding speech in noisy and/or reverberant environments. If the person also has tinnitus, it might seem logical to assume that the tinnitus is the cause of the speech understanding difficulties. Every time an adverse listening condition is encountered, the tinnitus gets blamed for any hearing difficulties. Over time, as the hearing loss progresses, increased attention is given to the tinnitus as the source of the listening problems. The frustrations that occur become associated with the tinnitus, such that even just thinking about the tinnitus can trigger negative reactions. This might be the point at which the patient encounters the clinician and states, "My tinnitus makes it difficult for me to hear." It is then incumbent upon the clinician to evaluate all of the available information, educate the patient about the true cause of the hearing difficulties, and prescribe appropriate treatment. In some cases, only the hearing loss requires treatment and hearing aids will remedy the problem. In other cases, even the use of adequate amplification will be insufficient to overcome the negative reactions associated with the tinnitus, and treatment specific to the tinnitus must be provided.

ADMINISTERING THE TRT INITIAL INTERVIEW

The following sections describe each step of administering the TRT Initial Interview, which is shown in Appendix A.

Patient Instructions

The TRT Initial Interview form starts with specific instructions for the patient. The instructions should be read aloud by the clinician to the patient to ensure that the patient has been properly informed of the functional differences between problems associated with "tinnitus," "sound tolerance," and "hearing." It is common for patients to confuse these three interrelated conditions; thus, the pre-interview instructions are essential. The Interview itself contains four sections: (1) Tinnitus (Questions 1-18), (2) Sound Tolerance (Questions 19-30), (3) Hearing (Questions 31-33), and (4) Ranking Problems (Questions 34-36).

The first five questions obtain descriptions of different parameters of the tinnitus percept. Although patients' responses to these questions have no bearing on how they will receive treatment, the information is important for a number of reasons. First, it is always necessary to provide descriptive information of the tinnitus symptom in clinical reports. Also, patients generally appreciate the opportunity to describe the sound that only they can hear to a sympathetic and understanding clinician. Further, the baseline description will be referred to at later appointments to determine if any tinnitus characteristics have changed during treatment. Changing the tinnitus percept is not a specific objective of treatment with TRT. Interestingly, however, it has been reported that approximately 20% of a group of 149 patients experienced a reduction or elimination of their tinnitus during treatment with TRT (Sheldrake, P. J. Jastreboff, & Hazell, 1996). Twenty-eight of these patients could not hear their tinnitus even when attempting to listen to it. The average period of time for this to occur was about 10 days. Although this kind of outcome is a possibility, it should not be mentioned to patients because of the potential of raising false expectations. The clinician should, however, be aware of this possibility and determine if these changes take place during treatment.

Question 1. What does your *most bothersome* tinnitus sound like?

Meikle et al. (1984) provided data from a large number of tinnitus patients from the Oregon Health & Science University Tinnitus Clinic, revealing that almost half of the patients reported that their tinnitus percept consisted of more than one distinct sound. Patients with "complex" tinnitus reported 2–5 different sounds. For TRT it is essential that patients identify the single sound that is considered to be the "most bothersome." According to the Meikle et al. data (which have been updated at http://www.tinnitusarchive.org), about half of tinnitus patients will experience multiple sounds (Meikle et al., 2004).

The patient's most bothersome tinnitus will be referenced often during the assessment and during treatment. The tinnitus psychoacoustic assessment includes matching the most bothersome tinnitus to external tones and attempting to suppress it with broadband noise. Treatment focuses on facilitating habituation to the most bothersome tinnitus. Patients who use ear-level sound generators or combination instruments must daily adjust the acoustic noise signal using the most bothersome tinnitus as the auditory reference (described in Chapter 13).

Question 2. Where is the location of your *most bothersome* tinnitus?

After patients have identified their most bothersome tinnitus, they are asked to describe its perceived location with respect to the head and/or ears. According to the Tinnitus Archive (Meikle et al., 2004), about 30% of patients report that their predominant tinnitus is perceived in one location, and 70% report multiple locations. Table 10–1 shows the tinnitus locations that were reported by these patients. (The data in Table 10–1 include both patients who reported a single tinnitus location as well as those who reported multiple locations.) The majority of patients (63%) reported that their tinnitus was perceived in "both ears." Thirteen percent perceived their tinnitus to be in their left ear, and 10.8% perceived it to be in the right ear. Another 11.4% reported that their tinnitus sound filled their head. Numerous additional perceived locations were reported by these patients.

TABLE 10–1. Perceived location of tinnitus, based on a sample of 1,629 patients evaluated at the OHSU Tinnitus Clinic. These data include patients who reported a single location as well as those who reported multiple locations for their tinnitus. Thus the percentages add up to greater than 100%. (From *Tinnitus archive* (2nd ed.), by M. B. Meikle, T. A. Creedon, & S. E. Griest, 2004. Retrieved April 29, 2004, from http://www.tinnitusarchive.org/.)

Location	N	Percent of 1,629 Patients
Both ears	1,026	63.0
Left ear	212	13.0
Inside head—left	91	5.6
Outside head—left	9	0.6
Not sure—left	2	0.1
Right ear	176	10.8
Inside head—right	80	4.9
Outside head—right	11	0.7
Fills head	186	11.4
Inside top of head	22	1.4
Outside top of head	3	0.2
Surrounds head	5	0.3
Back of head	49	3.0
Other answer	96	5.9

Question 3. Is your tinnitus louder on one side of your head than the other?

When asked about the location of their "worst" tinnitus, only about 25% of the OHSU Tinnitus Clinic patients reported that their tinnitus was symmetrical (Meikle et al., 2004). About 40% of the patients reported their worst tinnitus in their left ear, and about 32% in their right ear. For the TRT Initial Interview, there are only three possible response options: right louder than left, left louder than right, or equal (symmetrical).

Question 4. Is your tinnitus a constant sound or an intermittent sound?

Question 4 can be difficult for patients to answer because they often confuse periods of not being aware of their tinnitus with the tinnitus being absent altogether. Technically, the question's intent is to determine if, in a quiet environment, the tinnitus would be present all of the time ("constant") or only part of the time ("intermittent"). Patients are often unaware that background noise can suppress their tinnitus. Thus, the tinnitus could be constant but suppressed periodically by environmental sound. It has been shown that, using broadband noise, tinnitus can be completely suppressed within 3 dB Sensation Level (dB SL, i.e., level above hearing threshold) for 20% of patients, within 6 dB SL for 42% of patients, and within 12 dB SL for 70% of patients (Meikle et al., 2004). These data reveal that tinnitus is easily masked for many patients. This observation, however, is not consistent with other reports (e.g., Penner, Brauth, & Hood, 1981) and the common observation that patients with clinically significant tinnitus perceive it the majority of the time, even when they are in a relatively loud environment. The observation by Penner et al.—that it is necessary for many patients to increase the level of suppressing sound by as much as 45 dB when attempting to mask their tinnitus for 30 minutes—may help to explain these discrepant findings. For patients whose tinnitus is easily masked, there may be the perception that the tinnitus is intermittent when in fact it is only being suppressed during the "quiet" periods of tinnitus silence. If there is concern about the patient's understanding of the question's intent, the question can be rephrased as: "In a quiet environment, such as the one we are in now, if you listen for your tinnitus will you always hear it?"

Question 5. Does the loudness of your tinnitus change on its own?

Fluctuations in the perceived loudness of tinnitus are normal for most tinnitus patients. However, it is important for patients to distinguish between spontaneous changes in tinnitus loudness versus changes in loudness that result from variations in the auditory environment. Regarding the latter effect, the perceived loudness of tinnitus is often inversely related to the amount of ambient sound (Vernon, 1992). Patients thus might mistake these environment-induced changes in perceived loudness to be naturally-occurring changes. The intent of the question is to determine if there are changes in loudness that are not caused by external factors. If the patient reports natural fluctuations, the next part of the question then asks, "How often?" Fluctuations may occur multiple times during a single day, or they may occur more gradually over days or weeks. From a group of 745 patients in the Tinnitus Archive (Meikle et al., 2004), almost half reported that their tinnitus fluctuates daily. Only 10% reported that fluctuations were a rare occurrence. According to these data, it would be expected that most patients would report loudness fluctuations.

Patients are generally very aware of increases in tinnitus loudness, and they often report that their tinnitus is the most bothersome during these periods. Some patients report that there are observable patterns in their tinnitus fluctuations. The tinnitus is often reported to be louder when waking up in the morning. Some patients report that their tinnitus becomes louder as the day progresses. These would be considered "spontaneous fluctuations." Patients also report that their tinnitus becomes louder after being exposed to certain sounds, eating certain foods, being under extreme stress, being sleep deprived, etc. Loudness changes that occur as a result of these kinds of factors would not be considered spontaneous fluctuations. Increased loudness that results from exposure to certain sounds is addressed specifically in Question 8.

Question 6. Please describe the onset of your tinnitus.
How long have you had your tinnitus?

The first of these two questions determines whether patients noticed the onset of their tinnitus as "sudden" or "gradual." There are two reasons why this information can be helpful. First, sudden-onset tinnitus is often associated with a specific event, which may be important diagnostically. Second, knowing the circumstances of the tinnitus onset can help to explain why a patient's tinnitus became problematic. This kind of information addresses the root cause of the problem, both physiologically and psychologically. If a physiological cause can be determined, it is possible that the cause is amenable to medical or surgical intervention. If a psychological cause is apparent, this information can be useful for counseling purposes. With regard to counseling, it is often the case that a patient's tinnitus is associated with some stressful or traumatic event. When such an association is created, conscious attention given to the tinnitus can evoke memories of the emotion-inducing event, thereby triggering the same emotions (Chapter 6 describes this process in detail). Problematic tinnitus by definition causes activity in emotional centers of the brain (Chapter 4). Obtaining information about what precipitated the emotional activity, however, can make the counseling more focused and more efficient. It should be noted that up to one-half of tinnitus patients are unable to associate their tinnitus onset with a causal event. According to the Tinnitus Archive (Meikle et al., 2004), 43% of tinnitus patients could not identify any "illness, accident, or other special circumstances" that were associated with their tinnitus onset.

Hazell (1996a) refers to causes of tinnitus as "trigger factors," and divides them into four groups: ear related, psychological trauma, physical trauma, and unknown. Hazell states "psychological or stress-related events are far more powerful triggers for tinnitus onset than ear-related events" (p. 56). Thus, while there may be an identifiable physiological cause for the onset of tinnitus, it is more important to identify any psychological or stress-related events that triggered emotional reactions in response to the tinnitus. As an example, a person may have tinnitus that is a benign auditory signal causing no undue attention and no reactions. If the person experiences psychological trauma (which may be a period of depression, anxiety, or stress), the person's sensitivity to sensory stimuli may be heightened. The tinnitus neural signal is processed as a sensory stimulus, and the signal may become prominent as a result of the trauma. If the signal is interpreted as being threatening in any way, the brain will continue to monitor the signal as part of the survival mechanism (Hazell, 1996b). In this case a small signal has taken on emotional significance, with the net result that the tinnitus has gone from being a benign signal to becoming a continuous source of annoyance. The tinnitus may be perceived as louder, and the person pays much more attention to it. This scenario also can occur when there was no awareness of tinnitus. That is, a tinnitus neural signal may be present and yet completely undetectable in the auditory system. In this case the increased sensory sensitivity caused by the psychological trauma can cause the previously undetectable tinnitus signal to be detected and ultimately to become a source of distress.

The second of the two questions (How long have you had your tinnitus?) determines the length of time that the patient has been consciously aware of the continuous presence of tinnitus. An important concern is to determine the likelihood that the tinnitus will spontaneously resolve. Tinnitus of at least 6 months' duration is normally considered to be permanent with little chance of complete abatement. Tinnitus of recent onset (up to about 3 months' duration), however, is considered more labile with a greater probability of spontaneous resolution (Meikle, 1991b). All patients, especially those with recent-onset tinnitus, should be counseled to do everything possible to maximize any chance that the tinnitus will be reduced in intensity or disappear altogether. There is also the scenario described in the above paragraph whereby a benign tinnitus signal suddenly becomes intrusive as a result of some significant psychological event. The tinnitus signal may have been present for a long period, but the reactions to the signal might have started more recently. The most important consideration in counseling the patient is to provide positive information to dispel any fears or anxieties that have become associated with the tinnitus. It is often the case that some other medical practitioner gave the patient "negative counseling," meaning that the patient was told that the tinnitus is untreatable, that little is known about it, and that the only recourse is to "learn to live with it." Negative counseling occurs very commonly with tinnitus patients and can result in a greatly exacerbated condition. The TRT clinician must determine if this has occurred, and replace thoughts of hopelessness with an understanding that tinnitus is treatable, that much is known about it, and that there are many avenues that can lead to the tinnitus being processed as a benign signal.

Question 7. Do you have "bad days" when your tinnitus is more bothersome than usual, or does it seem equally bothersome from day to day?

Most patients can easily relate to the idea that there are certain days during which their tinnitus is particularly bothersome. This question asks if such bad days occur. If so, the question quantifies the response by asking how often bad days occur with respect to a week, a month, or a year. The patient's response provides a unique outcome variable that is a good indicator of treatment efficacy if the number of bad days decreases over time.

Question 8. Do sounds ever cause a change in the loudness of your tinnitus?

Question 8 addresses the primary issue that is critical to determining if a patient should be placed in Category 4. Category 4, as described in Chapter 9, is fairly uncommon and includes patients who experience prolonged exacerbation of tinnitus intensity when exposed to certain sounds that are not dangerously loud. The effect has been likened to *kindling* or *winding-up,* as also described in Chapter 9. Some patients may experience tinnitus exacerbation for minutes or for hours, but the tinnitus must remain louder until at least the following day to consider Category 4 placement. The exacerbation can occur for days or weeks. Patients in Category 4 are the most difficult to treat effectively, and extended treatment is probably indicated (P. J. Jastreboff, 1998, 1999a). The condition is almost always experienced by patients who predominantly have a hyperacusis problem (P. J. Jastreboff & Hazell, 2004). Treatment focuses on desensitization of auditory pathways, similar to treatment for hyperacusis.

A simple answer of "louder" from the patient is insufficient to make an automatic Category 4 placement decision. Question 8 therefore includes a series of additional questions. The patient answering "louder" is first asked, "What kinds of sounds cause this change?" The types of sounds that would likely be responsible for a tinnitus-exacerbation effect are listed. The clinician should not mention the items from this list, but rather should elicit answers from the patient in an open-ended way, i.e., without cues. Sounds that patients mention should fit one of the sound categories provided (there is also the category of "other"). When the responsible sounds have been identified, the clinician asks the patient how long the tinnitus-exacerbation effect lasts. Response boxes are provided to record the patient's answer. At this point the key question is asked, "Does the effect sometimes last until the next morning after you've slept?" If the patient answers "No," then it can be reasonably deduced that the patient does not have a sound-exacerbation problem, and Question 8 is complete. If the patient answers "Yes," then the patient is again asked what kinds of sounds cause the effect. The kinds of sounds that would cause this effect are again listed, which again should not be referred to when obtaining the patient's response. Any sounds that are identified in this last part of the question are very important for any counseling the patient might receive. It should be noted that some of the sounds listed might be sounds that cause damage to the auditory system. If only these louder sounds are the cause of the patient's tinnitus-exacerbation problem, then the patient should be counseled to protect his or her ears from such sounds. It is thus possible that the exacerbation is actually caused by physiological damage, and would not be considered a kindling effect that would define Category 4. The possibility that a patient's response results from misophonia should also be considered.

Question 9. Do you use ear protection (earplugs or earmuffs)?

This question is the first of a series of questions that ultimately intend to determine if patients are *overprotecting* their ears. These questions follow naturally from the line of questioning in Question 8 that addresses the concern that tinnitus can be exacerbated by sound. Patients need to understand that loud sounds can cause damage and permanently exacerbate a tinnitus problem—thus necessitating the appropriate use of hearing protection. They also need to understand, however, that inappropriate use of hearing protection can greatly enhance the tinnitus problem. Some patients use earplugs or earmuffs because of their belief that certain sounds, or sound in general, will cause their tinnitus to become worse. They need to be educated that overuse of hearing protection can result in heightened sensitivity to sound, as well as the perception that the tinnitus is louder due to the occlusion effect (Formby & Gold, 2002; Formby, Sherlock, & Gold, 2002; Gold et al., 1999; Hazell & Sheldrake, 1992; McKinney, Hazell, & Graham, 1999; Vernon & Press, 1998; Wolk & Seefeld, 1999). If such overuse has already occurred, then it is important that the patient take steps to "undo" the process by gradually reducing the use of hearing protection. These patients must progress to the point that they only use hearing protection when exposed to sounds that can cause damage to the auditory system. When addressing these issues it is possible that patients who do not have this problem might acquire a new concern that sound can make their tinnitus worse. The examiner must be sensitive to this possibility and use care to prevent giving such an impression.

Question 10. Are you currently receiving any other treatment specifically for your tinnitus?

Many patients undergoing a tinnitus evaluation report that they have received different treatments for their tinnitus that have been ineffective. Some patients will also be receiving or self-administering treatment at the time of the examination. Most commonly these latter patients are taking a prescription drug or using some kind of dietary supplement. The point of the question is to determine if patients are receiving any kind of therapy currently that would conflict with TRT. With regard to medications and dietary supplements, none are consistently effective for tinnitus patients (Dobie, 1999; J. A. Henry, Dennis, et al., 2005; P. J. Jastreboff & Hazell, 2004). Patients should be counseled about this, but any change in a drug regimen should be made only under the supervision of the dispensing physician.

The use of benzodiazepines is known to impair neural plasticity (Kilic, Curran, Noshirvani, Marks, & Basoglu, 1999; Verwey, Eling, Wientjes, & Zitman, 2000; Ziemann, Hallett, & Cohen, 1998), which could potentially retard, or even counteract, habituation. However, patients have been known to habituate appropriately when using low doses of benzodiazepines, especially during the early stages of treatment. This being said, clinicians should not disqualify patients from initiating TRT solely on the basis of their concomitant benzodiazepine use. Benzodiazepines can be tapered slowly to zero without rebound tinnitus increases and/or regression of habituation.

Question 11. What is the *biggest reason* your tinnitus is a problem (not including trouble hearing or trouble understanding speech)?

Tinnitus questionnaires generally provide prompts to patients by referring to specific issues that might be impacted by tinnitus. For each question, patients check a box or provide a number that indicates the level of impact regarding the particular issue described in the question. Questionnaires, however, are limited to relatively few concerns that may not include the patient's *primary* problem that is ascribed to the tinnitus. Tinnitus clinicians are aware of the multidimensional aspect of tinnitus effects, and a list of these effects could include "thousands" of items (Tyler, 1993, p. 378). Question 11 is therefore intentionally open-ended to allow patients to express, without any prompting, the primary reason their tinnitus is a problem. A patient's response to this question should reveal the main objective of the treatment. The question specifically includes the wording, "not including trouble hearing or trouble understanding speech," to ensure that the response is not confounded by the (usually erroneous) perception that hearing difficulties are caused by the tinnitus.

Question 12. I'm going to read through a list of activities and I want you to tell me how often your tinnitus keeps you from doing these activities, or how often it negatively affects these activities in any way. Please don't include trouble hearing or trouble understanding speech when you answer these questions.

The previous Question 11 allows patients to express openly why they believe their tinnitus is a problem. While it is important to obtain unrestricted responses from patients, it is also important to mention specific problems that are commonly reported by tinnitus patients. Patients can always report the primary reasons they are bothered by their tinnitus. They generally cannot, however, provide a detailed list of life activities that are adversely affected by their tinnitus. Question 12 provides such a list, and patients are asked *how often* their tinnitus affects each activity.

Although not comprehensive, the activities mentioned are representative of the kinds of problems that are reported most often by tinnitus patients. The combined responses to the different activities reveal a profile of the impact of tinnitus on the patient's life, and indicate the areas that the treatment program should be successful in resolving. Patients are again reminded to refer specifically to activities affected by tinnitus and not by a hearing problem.

Question 13. What percent of your *total awake time*, over the last month, were you *noticing*, or *thinking about*, your tinnitus? Please give an average percentage over the last month.
Question 14. What percent of your *total awake time*, over the last month, were you *annoyed, distressed*, or *irritated* by your tinnitus? Please give an average percentage over the last month.

In Part 1 of this book, the concepts of consciousness and directed attention were discussed. These concepts are relevant to Question 13, which asks patients to report the percentage of time that their tinnitus is part of their consciousness or receives their directed attention. Reducing this percentage is the secondary objective of TRT (habituation of tinnitus *perception*). Question 14 addresses the primary objective of TRT, which is to reduce the percentage of time that patients are annoyed by their tinnitus (habituation of tinnitus *reaction*). To respond to each of these two questions, patients are asked to estimate the average percentage of time over the previous month. If the treatment is fully successful these percentages will drop to zero or close to zero at later appointments.

When asking Question 14, the examiner must be aware that emotional responses can occur even when there is no conscious awareness of the situation that has caused the emotion (as explained by conditioned reflexes—see Chapter 4). Physical emotional states can be produced entirely by subconscious processing—a concept that is critical for the proper implementation of TRT (see also Nonconscious Learning in Chapter 6). Patients responding to this question thus need to be instructed that their emotional state is partially affected by subconscious reactions. (This concept is addressed more directly by Question 16.) When they later receive counseling, they will learn that reactions of the sympathetic part of the autonomic nervous system cause tinnitus to become clinically significant. Even if they are aware of limited emotional responses, they may have very strong autonomic responses.

Question 15. How *strong*, or *loud*, was your tinnitus, on average, over the last month? "0" would be "no tinnitus"; "10" would be "as loud as you can imagine."
Question 16. How much has tinnitus *annoyed you*, on average, over the last month—not including annoyance from trouble hearing or trouble understanding speech? "0" would be "not annoying at all"; "10" would be "as annoying as you can imagine."
Question 17. How much did tinnitus *impact your life*, on average, over the last month—not including impact from trouble hearing or trouble understanding speech? "0" would be "not at all"; "10" would be "as much as you can imagine."

Each of these three questions asks essentially the same thing but from a different perspective. They all refer indirectly to the *severity* of tinnitus, i.e., the degree to which tinnitus impacts quality of life (J. A. Henry, Dennis, et al., 2005). While it may seem obvious that annoyance (Question 16) and impact on life (Question 17) are clearly indicators of tinnitus severity, the perceived loudness of tinnitus (Question 15) may not be intuitively associated with tinnitus severity. However, ranking the loudness of tinnitus has been shown to be generally correlated with tinnitus severity (Kuk, Tyler, Russell, & Jordan, 1990; Meikle, 1991b). Patient data from the Tinnitus Archive (Meikle et al., 2004) reveal that about 85% of this large sample of tinnitus patients reported their perceived tinnitus loudness as 5 or more on a 0–10 loudness-rating scale (with 10 representing *very loud*). It should be noted that tinnitus loudness matches, as described in Chapter 11, do not correlate with tinnitus severity (J. A. Henry & Meikle, 2000).

Questions 15–17 all use an ordinal response scale of 0 to 10, and patients are asked to rank their tinnitus with respect to its loudness, annoyance, and impact on life. The endpoints of each scale are labeled, and patients are required to select a number between the two extremes. The rankings that patients provide at the intake appointment are particularly useful when assessing outcome of treatment.

Question 18. Do you have any other comments about your tinnitus?

Question 18 gives patients the opportunity to express any concerns about their tinnitus that might not have been mentioned to this point. In most cases the Interview questions will have addressed all of the issues and patients will have nothing further to add.

Question 19. Are sounds bothersome or unpleasant to you when they seem normal to other people around you?

This question initiates a series of questions that are specific to problems with decreased sound tolerance. If patients respond that sounds are not bothersome or unpleasant to them when they seem normal to other people, the remaining sound tolerance questions are skipped. It is thus critical that patients correctly interpret the meaning of Question 19. If they answer "Yes," then they are asked to indicate the kinds of sounds that cause the problem. A list of different categories of sounds is provided, but the examiner should not mention these different categories or any specific sounds so as not to lead the patient. If hypersensitivity to sound is truly a problem, patients know what kinds of sounds cause the problem. Completion of this question provides an inventory of sounds that are bothersome to the patient (P. J. Jastreboff & Hazell, 2004).

Question 20. Do these sounds cause you pain or physical discomfort?

Hypersensitivity to sound can involve the different components of hyperacusis, misophonia, and phonophobia (P. J. Jastreboff & M. M. Jastreboff, 2000). (Please refer to Chapter 9 for explanations of these conditions.) The questions about sound tolerance help to guide the patient and clinician to an understanding of which components are involved in the problem. While there may be subtle differences, it is important to make the correct diagnosis because treatment will differ depending on the specific condition (P. J. Jastreboff & Hazell, 2004). Question 20 specifically addresses hyperacusis, which is a physiological response to sound involving some level of physical discomfort. Patients with significant hyperacusis almost always also experience misophonia, especially those who have experienced hyperacusis for an extended period of time (M. M. Jastreboff & P. J. Jastreboff, 2002; P. J. Jastreboff & Hazell, 2004).

Question 21. Do you have "bad days" when sound tolerance is more of a problem than on other days, or is your ability to tolerate sound the same from day to day?

This is the same question as for Question 7, except that it is specific to a sound tolerance problem. Although less common than for tinnitus, some patients know that their sound tolerance problem is more bothersome on some days than others. If so, they are asked to indicate how often these bad days occur. Their responses to this question over the period of treatment provide a good measure of treatment efficacy.

Question 22. Do sounds ever cause a change in how much sound you can tolerate?

Question 22 is the sound tolerance version of Question 8, which was specific to tinnitus. Just as sound can exacerbate a tinnitus problem, it can also exacerbate a sound tolerance problem. Question 22 thus helps to determine if a patient should be placed in Category 4 because of hyperacusis. This category includes patients who experience prolonged worsening of sound sensitivity until at least the next morning when exposed to certain sounds (see Chapter 9). As for Category 4 as it pertains to tinnitus, successful outcome of treatment is less assured, and extended treatment may be necessary. Patients often have prolonged exacerbation to both tinnitus and sound sensitivity.

Question 22 includes a series of additional questions that are designed to obtain all of the information necessary to determine if Category 4 placement is appropriate. These questions are essentially the same as for Question 8 and the reader is referred to that question above for further elaboration. Importantly, the clinician should not mention the types of sounds that are listed in the Interview. Patients should volunteer this information, without being prompted, to obtain the most relevant responses.

Question 23. (Interviewer: In Question 9 did the patient report use of hearing protection because of "trouble tolerating everyday sounds"?) (IF YES) Earlier you told me that you sometimes use ear protection because of trouble tolerating sound—what percent of the time do you use ear protection *because of that trouble*?

In Question 9, patients were asked if they use hearing protection because of "trouble tolerating everyday sounds that seem normal to others." If the response to this question was negative, then Question 23 is passed over. If they reported this specific use of hearing protection, then the series of questions under Question 23 is asked. Question 9 is designed to determine if patients overprotect their ears to prevent their tinnitus from becoming worse. Similarly, Question 23 is designed to determine if there is overuse of hearing protection because of worries that sound will worsen a sound sensitivity problem. If this is the case, it is especially important to provide counseling that overuse of hearing protection can increase sensitivity to sound (Formby & Gold, 2002).

Question 24. Are you currently receiving any treatment specifically for problems with *sound tolerance*?

It is less likely that patients are receiving some other treatment for their sound tolerance problem than for a tinnitus problem. However, it is important to ask Question 24 to ensure that patients are not receiving or self-administering any kind of therapy that would either worsen their sound tolerance condition or potentially conflict with treatment they would receive with TRT.

Question 25. What is the major reason *trouble tolerating sound* is a problem?

Prior to reading through the list in Question 26 of potential reasons why sound tolerance is a problem, patients are asked to state *of their own accord* why sound tolerance is a problem. Their answer to this open-ended question indicates the primary objective of treatment.

Question 26. I'm going to read a list of activities and I want you to tell me how often trouble tolerating sound keeps you from doing these activities, or how often it negatively affects these activities in any way.

As for Questions 11 and 12, Questions 25 and 26 require patients to provide an open-ended answer for the main reason for their problem, followed by a list of common problems caused by the problem. Question 26 provides a list that is slightly different than that used for Question 12. The items listed in Question 26 are all common activities that can be affected by a sound tolerance problem. The clinician reads each item and asks the patient to indicate how often the activity is affected by the sound tolerance problem by responding *never*, *rarely*, *sometimes*, *often*, or *always* (or *N/A*). A profile of activities affected by sound hypersensitivity is created, and the relative rankings indicate the areas that are most affected. Successful treatment should modify the profile such that the different activities are affected "rarely" or "never."

Question 27. Please rate your *ability to tolerate sound* on a scale of "0" to "10." "0" would mean "you can tolerate all sounds"; "10" would mean "you cannot tolerate any sounds."

Question 28. How much has trouble tolerating sound *annoyed you*, on average, over the last month? "0" would be "not annoying at all"; "10" would be "as annoying as you can imagine."

Question 29. How much did trouble tolerating sound *affect your life*, on average, over the last month? "0" would be "not at all"; "10" would be "as much as you can imagine."

Each of these questions addresses a different aspect of severity of a sound tolerance problem. For each question, patients are asked to indicate the number between 0 and 10 that best represents the degree of difficulty caused by the sound tolerance problem. The response numbers should be similar across the three questions.

Question 30. Do you have any other comments about *trouble tolerating sound*?

This final question in the sound tolerance section should involve the elicitation of any further information from patients that is necessary in determining the specific characteristics of their sound tolerance problem. Because of the potential difficulty in teasing apart effects of hyperacusis, misophonia, and phonophobia, the clinician should pursue this course of questioning until a clear diagnosis is obtained.

Question 31. Do you think you have a hearing problem?
Question 32. Have you ever worn hearing aids?
Question 33. Has anyone ever suggested that you try hearing aids?

Category 2 patients require hearing aids as part of their treatment with TRT. Hearing aids are used primarily as sound therapy for their tinnitus, while any improvement in communication skills is a secondary objective (P. J. Jastreboff & Hazell, 2004). The determination of need for hearing aids is based primarily on patients' subjective feelings about their need for amplification to assist them with their hearing; i.e., it is not a decision based solely on the audiogram. Asking these three questions can assist in making this determination. By this point in the Interview, patients should have a clear understanding of the relationship between their tinnitus and any hearing difficulties that they experience. Thus, they should not confuse the two when answering this question. However, some patients will continue to insist that their hearing problem is caused by their tinnitus. It is important for the clinician to be aware of this common misconception and to counsel accordingly (Coles, 1995; Dobie, 2004b; Zaugg et al., 2002).

Question 34. How much of a problem is *tinnitus* (if you are not including problems from trouble hearing or trouble understanding speech)? "0" would be "no problem at all"; "10" would be "as much as you can imagine."
Question 35. How much of a problem is *trouble tolerating sound*? "0" would be "no problem at all"; "10" would be "as much as you can imagine."
Question 36. How much of a problem is *hearing*? "0" would be "no problem at all"; "10" would be "as much as you can imagine."

These are the final questions in the Initial Interview, and they are designed to provide comparative rankings of the three potential auditory problems experienced by patients. Administering the Interview should have fully informed patients as to the differences between tinnitus, decreased sound tolerance, and hearing loss—differences that are surprisingly difficult for many patients to comprehend. Asking these questions side by side reveals the relative difficulties caused by the different problems. Of course not all patients will experience more than one problem, and only the relevant questions are asked. The responses should provide the final information needed to determine which patient category is most appropriate. If "trouble tolerating sound" is reported as the predominant problem, then the patient should be treated initially for the specific sound tolerance problem. Treatment should reduce this problem, whereby the tinnitus may emerge as the predominant problem.

The TRT Follow-up Interview (Chapter 14 and Appendix B) should be administered at each subsequent treatment appointment, which will provide these relative rankings that often shift over time. The TRT Follow-up Interview duplicates those questions from the TRT Initial Interview that would be considered necessary to monitor treatment progress and to determine treatment outcomes (M. M. Jastreboff & P. J. Jastreboff, 1999). Some of these questions have been modified relative to the Initial Interview as appropriate for follow-up evaluation.

11

Audiometric Testing

In addition to the Initial Interview, the assessment of patients for treatment with TRT involves audiometric testing, including an audiological assessment, psychoacoustic measures of tinnitus, and measures of loudness discomfort levels (LDLs) (P. J. Jastreboff, 2000). The audiometric tests listed below (in Order of Testing) are recommended for a comprehensive assessment. However, the only tests that are required to determine patient category and to initiate treatment are pure tone hearing thresholds, speech discrimination, and LDLs (P. J. Jastreboff & Hazell, 2004). An audiogram and speech discrimination scores are necessary to determine the extent of any hearing loss, while LDLs help to define a sound tolerance problem. All of the other tests would be considered useful in some way, but not necessary. The complete testing protocol described below allows the clinician to make a thorough assessment of the auditory system with respect to hearing function, sound tolerance, and tinnitus.

The psychoacoustic measurements of tinnitus are not diagnostic and will not influence the course of treatment, but they are important for several reasons (J. A. Henry, M. M. Jastreboff, et al., 2002). First, the test results are useful for counseling purposes. Second, these measures will be required if patients pursue legal action related to their tinnitus. Third, as argued elsewhere (J. A. Henry, Flick, Gilbert, Ellingson, & Fausti, 2004), quantification of symptoms is fundamental within any branch of medicine. With regard to this latter point, valid and reliable quantification of tinnitus perceptual attributes promotes efforts to (a) elucidate and diagnose underlying mechanisms of tinnitus, (b) design treatment that addresses specific tinnitus characteristics, and (c) determine effects of tinnitus upon its perceptual attributes.

ORDER OF TESTING

Comprehensive audiometric testing includes the following measures (listed in the recommended order of testing).

1. Pure tone hearing thresholds (0.125–12 kHz)
2. Speech recognition thresholds
3. Most comfortable listening level (MCL) for speech
4. Loudness discomfort level (LDL) for speech
5. Minimum suppression level (MSL)
6. Speech discrimination (at MCL)
7. Tinnitus loudness and pitch matching
8. LDLs to white noise and pure tones (0.5, 1, 2, 3, 4, 6, 8, and 12 kHz)
9. Distortion-product otoacoustic emissions (DPOAE)
10. Impedance audiometry (reflex and reflex decay testing are not normally advised)

In general, the audiological tests are performed as for any standard assessment of auditory function by an audiologist. Details of audiological tests are not described here, as they are available in any textbook of audiology. Since the tinnitus psychoacoustic tests are often not performed in a standardized manner, they will be described in some detail (see also J. A. Henry, 2004; J. A. Henry, M. M. Jastreboff, et al., 2002; J. A. Henry, Zaugg, et al., 2005).

The precise order of testing is not critical. It is important, however, for the examiner to be aware of certain concerns that can influence the testing. First, psychoacoustic tinnitus measures can be affected by the prior presentation of supra-threshold levels of sound (J. A. Henry, 2004). This would be due generally to the effect of *residual inhibition* (RI). A digression is necessary to explain RI. The clinical test for RI involves the presentation of 1 minute of broadband noise at a level 10 dB above the level of noise that just suppresses the tinnitus (Vernon & Meikle, 1988). If the tinnitus is reduced or rendered inaudible following the noise presentation, then the test is positive for RI. When tested in this manner, 80–90% of patients experience some degree of RI (J. A. Henry & Meikle, 2000; Vernon & Meikle, 2000). The RI effect is an objective of treatment with the method of Tinnitus Masking, but not with TRT. RI testing is therefore not included in the TRT assessment. Experiencing the RI effect can cause TRT patients to become confused regarding the objectives of treatment. With TRT, sound therapy requires that the patient's tinnitus perception remain unchanged to enable habituation to occur to the "usual" tinnitus (see Chapter 6). Patients are told that treatment will probably have no effect on their tinnitus, although clinical data have shown that some patients treated with TRT do experience a reduction in their tinnitus loudness (Sheldrake et al., 1996).

Audiometric testing exposes patients to many types of sounds, any of which can potentially induce RI (J. A. Henry, M. M. Jastreboff, et al., 2002). With the occurrence of RI, the patient's tinnitus perception changes, which can affect the tinnitus psychoacoustic measures. Some patients even report that they can't hear their tinnitus during or immediately after audiometric testing (indicating that complete RI has occurred). For these reasons it has been recommended that tinnitus matches (loudness and pitch) be obtained prior to the presentation of any supra-threshold sounds (J. A. Henry, Zaugg, et al., 2005). However, the recommended order of audiometric tests for TRT places tinnitus matching after some of the suprathreshold testing, which is acceptable because the results of tinnitus matching have no influence on treatment procedures with TRT (J. A. Henry, M. M. Jastreboff, et al., 2002; P. J. Jastreboff & Hazell, 2004).

A second issue that can affect testing is the common observation that many tinnitus patients also have decreased sound tolerance. In Chapter 9 the various aspects of a reduced sound tolerance problem were discussed. Regardless of how patients are affected by this problem, a basic premise of performing the audiometric assessment is that *a sound tolerance problem is assumed until testing proves otherwise* (P. J. Jastreboff & Hazell, 2004). Evaluation of tonal LDLs provides a reasonable estimate of the upper limit of the auditory dynamic range at the different audiometric frequencies. Prior to performing any audiometric testing, it would be optimal to know a patient's loudness discomfort levels (LDLs) so as not to exceed them during testing. However, LDL testing should not be performed first due to other considerations.

LDL testing can be an uncomfortable experience for some patients, especially for those who are phonophobic. These patients need to have a positive experience with audiometric testing prior to being tested with sounds that may cause discomfort. (Note that the instructions for LDL testing below are explicit in asking patients to report when the sounds reach a level that they would not want to listen to for more than a few seconds. The LDLs obtained in this manner are *at or just below* the level of discomfort.) Testing LDLs too early in the process can cause emotional reactions in patients. These negative reactions are highly undesirable in that patients can lose confidence in the examiner, which would undermine any efforts to instill a sense of trust. A positive patient-clinician relationship is absolutely vital to achieve optimal results from treatment.

It was explained above how LDL testing prior to obtaining tinnitus measures can affect the tinnitus measures (due to the potential of causing residual inhibition). Although not a major concern, the clinician should be aware of this potential.

The recommended testing order represents a compromise that is appropriate for performing a TRT assessment. Hearing and speech thresholds are tested first, followed by most comfortable listening level (MCL) and LDL for speech.

Determining speech LDLs early in the assessment helps to minimize the possibility that patients would be exposed to sounds that would cause a sound tolerance reaction. Testing for tonal LDLs is one of the last tests. Testing for tonal LDLs, however, requires considerably more time and effort than for speech LDLs, and the testing can be very aversive to some patients. Tonal LDL testing should at least be conducted before DPOAE and immittance testing due to the greater likelihood of these latter tests presenting sounds that are uncomfortable to the patient.

SPEECH TESTING (THRESHOLDS, MCL, AND LDL)

Speech recognition thresholds, and MCL and LDL for speech, provide information quickly regarding the patient's overall hearing level and dynamic range (P. J. Jastreboff & Hazell, 2004). Testing is normally conducted in 5-dB steps, but smaller step sizes should be used if a sound tolerance problem was reported during the Initial Interview. Measuring LDLs for speech requires a minimal presentation of louder sounds to obtain an estimate of pure tone LDLs. This estimate is useful when conducting the subsequent tests to reduce the potential for presenting sounds at uncomfortable levels. Obtaining LDLs for speech early during the assessment thus enables the more extensive pure tone LDL testing to be conducted toward the end of the assessment.

MINIMUM SUPPRESSION LEVEL (MSL)

Minimum suppression level has usually been referred to in the literature as minimum masking level. P. J. Jastreboff and M. M. Jastreboff (2001) explained that psychoacoustic "masking" actually involves interaction of sound vibrations on the basilar membrane. Because tinnitus is defined as neural activity in the auditory pathways, psychoacoustic masking cannot technically occur with tinnitus. The effect normally referred to as masking is thus more correctly a process of "suppression" of neural activity.

The MSL is the minimum level of noise (or of any sound) required to make a person's tinnitus inaudible. As for tinnitus loudness and pitch matching, measures of MSL are irrelevant to the treatment of patients with TRT (P. J. Jastreboff & Hazell, 2004). Group measures of MSL have, however, been reported to correlate with outcomes of treatment (P. J. Jastreboff, Hazell, & Graham, 1994). For patients in that study who showed improvement with their tinnitus problem, MSLs were observed generally to decrease. Further, P. J. Jastreboff and Hazell (2004, Figure 4-13, p. 166) present data revealing a strong correlation between change in the MSL and treatment success.

MSL Procedures

White noise from an audiometer is used to obtain measures of MSL. As for tinnitus loudness matches, MSLs are reported in dB SL; thus, white noise auditory thresholds are required prior to obtaining MSLs. Patients vary widely in their MSLs. The majority of a large sample of patients at the OHSU Tinnitus Clinic were masked by noise less than 10 dB SL (Meikle et al., 2004). It is therefore appropriate to use 1-dB step sizes to obtain thresholds and MSLs using white noise. About 15% of patients could not be masked at any level (which may have been due to either a problem tolerating the noise or to equipment limitations).

Obtaining Noise Thresholds

White noise thresholds are obtained in each ear—first to the nearest 5 dB, then as precisely as the audiometer will allow. Testing for white noise thresholds uses the same procedures as described below for the high-resolution threshold testing that precedes tinnitus loudness matching. MSLs are measured following testing for white noise thresholds. MSL testing can be done either binaurally or monaurally, depending on whether patients have bilateral or unilateral tinnitus, respectively. Patients with bilateral tinnitus are tested with a binaural stimulus because it can be difficult to identify when complete suppression occurs in only one ear (or in one side of the head). Also, binaural sound is usually required to achieve complete bilateral suppression (J. A. Henry, Zaugg, et al., 2005). Patients with unilateral tinnitus are tested most efficiently with monaural noise. Some patients with unilateral tinnitus discover that tinnitus also exists in the contralateral ear when the unilateral tinnitus is completely suppressed.

Obtaining MSL Measures

Prior to testing for MSL, patients are instructed to identify the softest level of noise that completely suppresses their tinnitus (J. A. Henry, Zaugg, et al., 2005). Testing levels for the noise are adjusted upward relative to the noise thresholds. For binaural testing, the right and left ear outputs from the audiometer are locked to maintain the same level above threshold for both ears simultaneously. Stimulus presentation starts at the noise-threshold level and the noise is raised in 1-dB steps. Patients with bilateral tinnitus are told to report if the suppression occurs in one ear only (which would identify the MSL for that ear). When this occurs, noise is presented continuously at the MSL for that ear while the level in the contralateral ear continues to be raised until the tinnitus in that ear is also suppressed (which identifies the MSL for the contralateral ear).

If the patient's tinnitus is unilateral, then the noise is presented to the tinnitus ear only. The noise is raised in 1-dB steps above the threshold level until the tinnitus is suppressed in the test ear (MSL for that ear). When this occurs, the patient is asked if there is any tinnitus in the contralateral ear. If not, MSL testing is complete. If the patient reports the presence of tinnitus in the contralateral ear, then the noise is presented continuously at MSL in the tinnitus ear, while noise in the contralateral ear is raised in 1-dB steps above threshold until the tinnitus is completely suppressed in that ear also (MSL for contralateral ear).

TINNITUS LOUDNESS AND PITCH MATCHING

Tinnitus matching identifies the frequency and level of a tone that is reported to be the closest approximation to a patient's tinnitus percept. To obtain a match, the clinician presents pure tones to the patient systematically (adaptively) to gradually approach and then to match the tinnitus with one of the tones. Not all patients can provide an exact match, but most patients can, even when they describe their tinnitus as sounding more like noise than a tone.

The testing described below would be fairly routine for a tinnitus clinic, regardless of the method of treatment being used. TRT, however, places little emphasis on these measures; thus, the clinician can opt to shorten the testing even further. The description below provides a method to obtain a match between the patient's perceived tinnitus pitch and an audiometric pure tone. If the patient initially describes the tinnitus as sounding more "noisy" than "tonal," the clinician can use narrow-band noise or even white noise in the attempt to identify a sound that closely approximates the sound of the patient's tinnitus. All that would be required would be to obtain the patient's assent that the sound being presented sounds similar to the sound of the tinnitus, and then to determine the loudness of the stimulus (in dB SL) that matches the loudness of the tinnitus.

As already mentioned, results of tinnitus matching are useful primarily for counseling and do not influence the course of treatment with TRT in any way. Tinnitus patients often present with fears and anxieties about their tinnitus, which are generally unfounded. From a historical perspective, it is at the point of initial contact with a clinician that patients have too often received erroneous negative counseling consisting of statements such as, "There is nothing that can be done about your tinnitus—you're going to have to learn to live with it." A critical aspect of counseling is thus to "demystify" any negative concepts that have become associated with the tinnitus (P. J. Jastreboff, 2000). The tinnitus match quantifies what was previously an entirely subjective sensation, which alone can be helpful to the patient. In addition, the educational counseling protocol includes a depiction of the patient's tinnitus match on the audiogram, which generally reflects the tinnitus as being a "small" or "faint" signal. That is, the loudness match at the pitch-match frequency is usually only a few decibels above the patient's threshold (J. A. Henry & Meikle, 2000). Using the audiogram, it should be explained to the patient that the tinnitus signal is very faint in relation to common environmental sounds. This information can help to offset the perception of the tinnitus as "loud."

Procedures for obtaining tinnitus loudness and pitch matches have varied greatly between clinicians, and standardization is sorely needed. Vernon and Meikle (1981) described a detailed tinnitus-matching protocol that was used for many years in their clinic. Their method provides the basis for numerous variations of tinnitus matching procedures, but their exact method is time consuming and requires specialized instrumentation. The method we propose here has its roots in Vernon and Meikle's methodology, but with adaptations for clinical expediency. Our method has also been described in Henry, Zaugg, and Schechter (2005).

Considerations Prior to Testing

Some important considerations when conducting tinnitus matching are (a) Make sure that the patient understands the meanings of "loudness" and "pitch," (b) identify the "tinnitus ear" and the "stimulus ear," (c) present tones at levels that are close to the patient's perceived tinnitus loudness, and (d) try not to present any tones that exceed the loudness of the patient's tinnitus by any substantial amount.

When conducting tinnitus matching, it is essential that patients understand the distinction between loudness and pitch. Surprisingly, many patients confuse these two auditory concepts (Vernon & Fenwick, 1984). Prior to testing the clinician should query the patient about these terms and provide instruction as necessary. The concept of loudness can be demonstrated simply by making the voice louder and softer, and by referring to volume on a TV or radio. Pitch can be related to a piano keyboard or to the practicing of musical scales (do re mi . . .). If the patient is wearing earphones, the concepts can be demonstrated by presenting different levels and different frequencies with the audiometer. A specific guide for using an audiometer for this purpose has been published (J. A. Henry, Flick, Gilbert, Ellingson, & Fausti, 2001).

When patients perform the matching task, they must identify the most bothersome tinnitus and its location (as explained in Chapter 10). Subjective matching is done between the most bothersome tinnitus and each test tone. If the most bothersome tinnitus is asymmetrical, then the tinnitus ear is the side with the most bothersome tinnitus. If the most bothersome tinnitus is perceived as symmetrical, then either ear can be the tinnitus ear. To perform the matching task, it is essential that patients distinguish clearly between the tinnitus and the test tone. This can be accomplished most readily if the tinnitus and the tone are separated as much as possible, i.e., by performing contralateral testing (Vernon & Fenwick, 1984; Vernon & Meikle, 1981, 2003). For example, if the patient reports that the most bothersome tinnitus is perceived "in the left side of the head," then the tinnitus ear would be the left ear, and the stimulus ear would be the right ear. If the patient reports a centralized location of the most bothersome tinnitus, or if it is perceived as equivalent in each ear, then either ear can be used as the stimulus ear (except that if one ear has better hearing that ear should be the stimulus ear).

It was mentioned above that patients often confuse the concepts of loudness and pitch. Not only can they confuse the meanings of these terms, but they also can confuse the concepts when making judgments during pitch matching. Because of this potential confusion it is important to present tones at levels that are close to the patient's perceived tinnitus loudness. Suggested starting levels are 10–20 dB Sensation Level (dB SL, i.e., level above hearing threshold), at frequencies where hearing is normal, and 5–10 dB SL (or less) at frequencies where hearing is impaired. Specific instructions are provided below for maintaining the appropriate levels of test tones for pitch matching.

Finally, it is important during loudness and pitch matching that tones do not exceed the loudness of tinnitus by a substantial amount. As already mentioned, sound can induce residual inhibition (RI). If RI occurs, then the tinnitus being matched is not the tinnitus that is normally experienced. Also, higher levels, especially at the beginning of the audiometric testing, can conceivably exceed the patient's LDL. This latter possibility seems less likely than inducing RI with test tones; thus, it is recommended that LDLs be obtained after the tinnitus matching.

Obtaining a Tinnitus Loudness and Pitch Match

To reiterate, the method described here is a shortened version that allows testing to take place rapidly using a clinical audiometer. The absolute measures are not critical. By complying with the considerations described above, this method will provide reasonably accurate measures that will serve to quantify the sensation and accomplish the primary purpose of using the data for counseling.

Pitch Matching

Testing should start at a frequency that is perceived by the patient as well below the tinnitus pitch. For most patients a 1,000 Hz tone is appropriate as the starting tone. The 1,000 Hz tone is initially presented at 10–20 dB SL, and the clinician asks the patient if the tinnitus is louder or softer than the tone (J. A. Henry, Zaugg et al., 2005). The output is adjusted accordingly so that the tone is perceived to be at a level that approximates the loudness of the tinnitus. Once this level is established (without being overly precise), the clinician asks the patient if the tinnitus is higher or lower pitched than the tone. The 1,000 Hz tone is usually reported to be lower in pitch than the tinnitus. This procedure is repeated at adjacent octave frequencies, while continuing to maintain output levels that are approximately equal to the loudness of the tinnitus (patients should be instructed at the beginning of testing to report any tones that seem substantially louder or softer than the tinnitus). One of the octave frequencies should be identified as a "close match" to the tinnitus, and testing then continues in the same manner at adjacent interoctave frequencies.

It is well documented that repeated pitch matching results in matches that vary over 2–3 octaves (Burns, 1984; J. A. Henry et al., 2000; J. A. Henry, Flick, et al., 2004; J. A. Henry et al., 2001; J. A. Henry et al., 1999; Penner, 1983; Tyler & Conrad-Armes, 1983). It is therefore important to present the pitch-matched tone in comparison to tones that are an octave higher and an octave lower (assuming these frequencies do not exceed the test frequencies available with the audiometer). The patient's choice when making these comparisons is considered the final pitch match.

Loudness Matching

Once the tinnitus has been matched for pitch, then the same tone is used to determine the level of the tone that matches the loudness of the tinnitus. The loudness match should be reported in dB SL; thus, both a threshold and a loudness match are obtained at the pitch-match frequency.

Because loudness matches at the pitch-match frequency are usually less than 10 dB SL (Fowler, 1942; Graham & Newby, 1962; Reed, 1960), the loudness match should be obtained using the smallest dB step size available with the audiometer (1 dB if possible). First, a threshold is obtained using the usual down-10 dB, up-5 dB method (Carhart & Jerger, 1959). The tone is then presented 5 dB below the threshold and increased in 1-dB steps to obtain a more precise threshold. Using ascending 1-dB steps, the precise threshold should be confirmed (or an average should be taken between two responses that are close to each other). The patient is then instructed that the tone will be made louder in small steps, and the task is to find the loudness level of the tone that matches the loudness of the tinnitus. The tone is raised above the precise threshold in 1-dB steps until a loudness match is reported. The loudness matching should be repeated, and an average of the two responses represents the final loudness match at the pitch-match frequency.

Matching to Noise

When a pitch and loudness match have been obtained, an option is to conduct further testing to determine if the tinnitus sounds more like a tone or more like noise (as mentioned above, testing with noise can be the only testing performed for patients with noise-type tinnitus). The pitch match is presented (at the approximate loudness-matched level) and compared to narrow band noise centered at the pitch-match frequency (and also presented at approximately the tinnitus loudness level). Patients are asked which of the two stimuli sounds more like their tinnitus. If the tone is selected, then no further testing is necessary. If the noise is selected, then the narrow band noise can be compared to wide band noise. If either of the noise stimuli is selected, then a threshold and loudness match should be performed with the noise, same as for the pitch-matched tone.

LOUDNESS DISCOMFORT LEVELS

The loudness discomfort level (LDL) for a sound is the threshold level at which the sound becomes uncomfortably loud. For TRT, LDLs are measured at a series of audiometric frequencies. Each pure tone LDL determines the upper limit of the auditory dynamic range for the frequency tested (M. W. Skinner, 1988). The dynamic range is the range on the audiogram between hearing thresholds and LDLs. Sound can be tolerated comfortably within this range. The measurement of LDLs at pure tone frequencies provides information that is important in determining the patient's TRT category, and should corroborate the patient's responses to the sound tolerance questions in the Initial Interview (Chapter 10).

Patient Instructions

Patient instructions are essential to obtaining proper measures. Even a slight variation in the instructions can result in patients' interpreting the task differently and providing different responses accordingly (Punch, Joseph, & Rakerd, 2004). It is therefore suggested that patients always be instructed to report when they would "not want to listen to the tone for more than a few seconds." Test frequencies are ordered from lowest to highest and each tone is presented for 1-2 seconds. Each of the frequencies is tested in one ear, followed by the other ear.

LDL Testing Procedures

Ideally, LDLs should be measured at octave frequencies between 0.5 and 8 kHz (0.5, 1, 2, 4, and 8 kHz) and at the interoctave frequencies 3, 6, and 12 kHz.

Test tones should be presented in a manner that minimizes discomfort during testing. It is especially important to select starting levels at each test frequency that are well within the comfortable range. However, the starting levels must not be so low that testing efficiency is compromised. For each ear, the initial test frequency is 0.5 kHz. Normally, a starting level of 50 dB HL is appropriate at 0.5 kHz but should be even lower if a sound tolerance problem was reported during the Initial Interview. Each stimulus presentation is raised in 5-dB increments (1 dB if a sound tolerance problem was reported) until the patient indicates that the sound would not be comfortable to listen to for "more than a few seconds."

After the first LDL is obtained at 0.5 kHz, that LDL can serve as a guide for the initial presentation level at the next test frequency (1 kHz). In general, the starting level at each frequency should be about 20 dB below the previous frequency's LDL. For example, if the LDL at 0.5 kHz is 80 dB HL, the starting tone at 1 kHz should be about 60 dB HL. Testing LDLs requires skill to select starting levels appropriately, to test rapidly, and to maintain the patient's comfort throughout testing.

Studies have shown that patients often respond inconsistently when LDLs are repeated within a session (Beattie & Sheffler, 1981; Byrne & Dirks, 1996; Hawkins, Walden, & Montgomery, 1987). For that reason, LDLs are measured twice —first in each ear, and then the entire set of measurements is repeated. The second set of measurements is recorded as the pure tone LDL measures.

Measurement of LDLs at audiometric frequencies is not normally performed by most audiologists. These measures are necessary, however, to quantify a patient's reported hypersensitivity to sound (P. J. Jastreboff & M. M. Jastreboff, 2000). This is a commonly reported problem among tinnitus patients—clinics have reported up to 45% of their patients indicated some degree of decreased loudness tolerance (Coles, 1996; Gold et al., 1999; Hazell, 1999; P. J. Jastreboff, 2000). Fortunately, the condition is generally treatable, and even curable, provided treatment is administered appropriately. Baseline tonal LDLs quantify the problem and provide a benchmark to document improvement during therapy. Successful treatment would result in LDLs approaching levels close to 100 dB HL (Formby & Gold, 2002; Gold et al., 1999).

IMMITTANCE AND DPOAE TESTING

Tympanometry is tested as part of a routine audiological examination to evaluate middle ear function. Acoustic reflex testing, however, can be highly aversive to tinnitus patients, and this testing is generally not recommended for patients who are being evaluated for treatment with TRT. However, the testing can be performed if the LDL measures indicate that the stimulus tones will not produce discomfort, and if the patient understands that these tones can be quite loud. Reflex testing has been known to cause exacerbation of tinnitus, and extreme care must be used in considering its use.

DPOAE testing is an option for patients, and results of testing are used mainly for counseling purposes. During the counseling there is a specific discussion about outer hair cells. Having the results of DPOAE testing during this counseling section can be helpful to the patient. P. J. Jastreboff and Hazell (2004) suggest that this test be performed using primary tones at 65/55 dB SPL, in the frequency range of 0.5–12 kHz, and using 10 points per octave.

ASSIGNING PATIENTS TO TRT CATEGORIES

Following the Initial Interview and audiometric assessment, patients are assigned to one of the five TRT categories that were described in Chapter 9. Table 9–1 summarizes the criteria for assigning patient categories. There are essentially four questions that must be answered when assigning a category: (a) Does the patient have a significant subjective problem with tinnitus? (b) Does the patient have a significant subjective problem with hearing? (c) Does the patient have a significant subjective problem with sound tolerance? (d) Is the patient's tinnitus (or hyperacusis) exacerbated for a prolonged period (minimally overnight) by exposure to certain types of sounds?

Patients with minimally bothersome tinnitus (or with recent-onset tinnitus) do not normally warrant treatment with ear-level devices. For these Category 0 patients, an assessment and some basic educational counseling are usually all that are necessary for them to be satisfied that they do not require further rehabilitative efforts. These patients may benefit from further treatment, but the time, effort, and expense required may outweigh the benefit. Patients who agree to receive long-term TRT must be convinced of the value of proactively pursuing a program that can be time consuming and expensive. To possess this level of motivation, the tinnitus must have a significant detrimental effect on their lives.

As explained in Chapters 9 and 10, it has been our experience that many individuals with hearing loss and tinnitus attribute their hearing difficulties to their tinnitus. These individuals have the conscious perception of tinnitus and they experience hearing difficulties in certain situations. It thus might make sense to them that their tinnitus is the cause and hearing problems are the effect. When evaluated, these patients are usually discovered to have a typical high-frequency hearing loss that would make it difficult to hear in noisy situations. The loss may or may not be so extensive as to require amplification. If amplification is indicated, however, the fitting of hearing aids can be beneficial to their minimal tinnitus problem (Henry, Zaugg, et al., 2005; Searchfield, 2005). Category 0 patients, whether requiring amplification or not, should always be counseled about the beneficial effects of sound therapy.

Category 1 and Category 2 patients have a problem with their tinnitus to such a degree that a minimum of 1 year of treatment is warranted. The clinician must be astute in assessing the true degree of tinnitus difficulty that is experienced by the patient. This assessment is made through the process of administering the TRT Initial Interview (Chapter 10). Interview administration contains an important didactic component that requires the clinician to clearly explain the intent of each question. The accuracy of a patient's answers will be largely dependent upon this skill of the examiner. Both the patient and the clinician must be convinced that treatment is needed.

Category 2 patients have the further concern of significant hearing difficulties. The clinician must assess the differential effects of hearing loss and tinnitus, and both must be a significant problem to the patient for placement into Category 2.

The audiogram may suggest that amplification would be beneficial, but Category 2 placement is determined mainly by a patient's report of significant life problems induced by hearing difficulties. Category 2 patients will be fitted with amplification, usually in the form of a combination instrument—hearing aid plus sound generator. It is important that both the patient and the clinician understand that the primary purpose of amplification is to provide sound therapy for facilitating habituation to tinnitus. Thus, any improvement in hearing function is considered a secondary objective.

Category 3 patients have hyperacusis as the primary complaint. Technically, hyperacusis in the context of TRT is diagnosed on the basis of reduced LDLs, as defined above. However, patients' subjective impressions of loudness tolerance problems may or may not be consistent with their LDLs, and the combined data must be considered. Making an accurate assessment of this problem again requires skill on the part of the examiner. The TRT Initial Interview (Appendix A) contains an entire section about sound tolerance (Questions 19–30), which is generally sufficient to assess the extent of the problem. If the patient has a significant problem with hyperacusis, he or she should be assigned to Category 3 and treated accordingly.

It was explained in Chapter 9 how hyperacusis patients usually also have misophonia (that can be manifested as phonophobia). The treatments are dramatically different for hyperacusis and misophonia, while the same for misophonia and phonophobia. It is essential to counsel these patients appropriately for the different conditions (as described in Chapter 15).

Category 4 is reserved for patients who not only have a problem with tinnitus, but the further problem of extended tinnitus exacerbation as a consequence of exposure to certain sounds. The TRT Initial Interview (Appendix A) uses Question 8 to address this issue, and the patient's answers to this block of questions provide the critical information to determine if Category 4 placement is appropriate. Question 8 is specific to tinnitus exacerbation, but there is also the potential for patients to experience exacerbation of sound tolerance problems as a result of exposure to certain sounds. Prolonged exacerbation with respect to hyperacusis is addressed in Question 22, which contains a block of questions that are similar to Question 8. Category 4 patients comprise a small percentage of tinnitus and hyperacusis patients, but it is important to determine if prolonged exacerbation is an issue for patients so that they can receive proper treatment for the condition.

PART 3

Clinical Guidelines for Treatment

The purpose of Part 3 is to suggest guidelines for administering clinical treatment that is consistent with the principles of TRT. Part 3 includes (a) a description of how the TRT counseling protocol relates to different forms of psychological counseling (Chapter 12) (b) a specific script that models a complete TRT educational counseling session (Chapter 13) (c) clinical guidelines for ongoing treatment appointments (Chapter 14), and (d) guidelines for treatment of decreased sound tolerance (Chapter 15). There are of course variations in how TRT would be conducted according to a patient's treatment category and individual needs, but the main components of the protocol covered in Part 3 can be used as a general guide.

The TRT practitioner should have a clear understanding of the principles of treatment with TRT. These principles are described in detail in P. J. Jastreboff and Hazell (2004), and Part 1 of the present book provides material that supplements that seminal book for TRT. An overview of the main components of TRT is provided below

PURPOSE OF TRT COUNSELING

TRT uses a structured educational-counseling protocol as its most critical component of treatment (P. J. Jastreboff, 2000). The counseling is based strictly on the neurophysiological model of tinnitus. The information conveyed to patients is quite technical, and requires intensive teaching sessions. The presumption is that tinnitus, at the neurophysiological level, is a neural signal capable of affecting systems in the brain that are responsible for emotional and autonomic reactions. For the distressed patient, the tinnitus neural signal is classified by brain processing mechanisms as an important stimulus that requires continual monitoring. The stimulus is classified in this way if it is identified as aversive or threatening, or because it triggers negative emotional memories. A positive feedback loop of monitoring the signal and reacting to it is established, and the signal and its functional links with the limbic and autonomic nervous systems must be manipulated in some way to break this cycle. The TRT counseling information is intended to facilitate a reclassification of the tinnitus signal by these processing mechanisms to the category of an inconsequential stimulus. This process of reclassification is accomplished by providing the patient with a clear, coherent explanation of mechanisms that underlie the generation of tinnitus perception and the governing of tinnitus-induced distress. Successful counseling will remove negative associations with the tinnitus. These negative associations need to be removed for habituation to occur (P. J. Jastreboff & Hazell, 1998).

PURPOSE OF TRT SOUND THERAPY

Whereas the counseling for TRT addresses conscious levels of thought and the associated emotional responses, sound therapy is intended to modify auditory processing at primarily subconscious levels. The neural changes induced by sound therapy facilitate habituation to the tinnitus signal. Sound therapy cannot be effective in facilitating habituation unless the counseling is successful in removing negative associations with the tinnitus. It is for this reason counseling is considered the most important component of treatment with TRT.

Nonetheless, treatment with TRT always includes sound therapy, which may or may not involve the use of ear-level devices (P. J. Jastreboff, 2000; P. J. Jastreboff & M. M. Jastreboff, 2000). During TRT counseling, patients are instructed about the concepts of sound therapy, including the necessity to avoid silence and to maintain an "enriched" sound environment. This counseling is done with all patients, regardless of their treatment category, to the degree necessary for them to understand and to implement the essential principles of sound therapy.

Category 0 patients do not have tinnitus of such severity as to warrant the purchase and use of ear-level sound generators. Patients with more severe tinnitus (i.e., patients in categories other than Category 0) are advised to obtain ear-level devices (sound generators, hearing aids, or combination instruments) and to use them as directed in conjunction with a series of treatment sessions that will last typically 1 year. These patients must therefore appreciate the value of using ear-level devices and be motivated and committed to comply with the total treatment protocol. They should be counseled on the benefits of pairing the tinnitus percept with a benign, neutral, and therapeutic wide-band sound signal. The signal should be delivered from ear-level devices during all waking hours, at a level at or below the perceived "mixing point" (as explained in Chapter 13). All patients are instructed to enrich their auditory background by using table-top sound machines and other means of providing augmentative sound. This is particularly crucial for patients with hearing loss who are using hearing aids. The proper implementation of sound therapy ultimately facilitates habituation of tinnitus perception.

12

Principles of TRT Counseling

There has been considerable confusion and debate concerning the approach to counseling that is used with TRT (M. M. Jastreboff, 1999; McKenna, 2004; Wilson, 2006; Wilson, J. L. Henry, Andersson, Hallam, & Lindberg, 1998). There are numerous aspects to this debate, one of which is the "directive" style of counseling that has been advocated for TRT. It is therefore important to explain what is meant by directive counseling within the context of administering treatment with TRT.

NONDIRECTIVE VERSUS DIRECTIVE COUNSELING

Hodgson (1994a) noted that there are two major areas of counseling: emotional support and communication of information. Similarly, Clark and Martin (1994) noted a clear division between emotional support counseling and content-educational counseling. These two approaches to counseling can be referred to as *nondirective* and *directive*, respectively. Nondirective counseling is also known as client-centered therapy, meaning that the emphasis of counseling is on the patient more than on the problem. The goal of client-centered therapy is for patients to experience "growth," which enables them to be better equipped to deal with future problems. Patients are encouraged to share their thoughts and beliefs with the counselor who affirms their worth by listening. Ultimately, nondirective counseling is a technique whereby the counselor leads the patient in the self-realization of solutions.

In its strictest sense, directive counseling has little in common with the nondirective approach of leading patients gradually in the self-discovery of solutions. Directive counseling focuses on the problem that is the reason for therapy. The goal is to solve the problem through the provision of new information and attitudes to the patient. The clinician determines the goal of treatment, and assists the patient in attaining that goal.

DIRECTIVE COUNSELING IN RELATION TO PSYCHOLOGICAL FORMS OF THERAPY

To understand the concepts of directive counseling, it is important to understand the different psychological forms of counseling and how they are adapted for treatment of tinnitus. Clark and Martin (1994) noted that patients with auditory problems (specifically, audiology patients) are generally psychologically-normal people who by definition would not require psychotherapy. This view is corroborated by J. L. Henry and Wilson (1998, p. 34) who state, "The vast majority of people who are troubled by their tinnitus do not display clear-cut psychiatric disorders but are, nevertheless, distressed and impaired by the tinnitus." Counseling of these patients would thus remain primarily in the content realm, and emotional support counseling would be limited to helping them to make practical, positive changes in their lives. In the context of the tinnitus patient who is "psychologically normal," there are three counseling theories with which clinicians should be familiar. These three theories are described briefly below.

Rogers' Person-Centered Counseling

Person-centered counseling defines the pure nondirective approach as originally espoused by Carl Rogers. As mentioned above, nondirective counseling focuses on the patient more than on the problem. With this approach, "the patient knows best" (Clark & Martin, 1994). The clinician avoids any appearance of being the expert who will provide specific solutions, but rather serves as a facilitator to challenge patients to accept the responsibility of finding "inner resources" to solve their own problems. It is important for the clinician to exhibit to the patient an "unconditional positive regard" and an "empathic understanding" so as to positively reinforce the patient's self-directed efforts.

Behavioral Counseling Theory

In Chapter 6, classical conditioning is contrasted with instrumental conditioning. Most basically, with classical conditioning an association is learned between two stimuli. With instrumental conditioning, an association is learned between a behavior and a consequence. Instrumental conditioning (also referred to as *operant conditioning* and *trial-and-error learning*) was originally defined by J. Konorski in 1932 and published in English in 1948 (Konorski, 1948). B. F. Skinner (1953), the leading proponent of instrumental conditioning, defined it as the increased probability of performing a behavior when it is learned that the behavior brings satisfaction (Clark & Martin, 1994).

To use behavioral counseling, the clinician guides the patient through a series of "successive approximations" (incremental behavioral changes) that lead toward the desired goal (Clark & Martin, 1994). The approach is thus primarily directive rather than nondirective, although supportive aspects of person-centered counseling can be combined with behavioral counseling to enhance its effectiveness.

Cognitive Counseling Theory

Cognitive forms of therapy address "irrational thoughts and beliefs" that cause self-defeating behaviors (Clark & Martin, 1994). These thoughts and beliefs are brought to conscious awareness as the patient is led through a process of analyzing the relationships between cognitions, emotions, and events (Wilson, 2006). Strategies for achieving the goals of cognitive therapy include direct questioning of stated assumptions (challenging cognitive distortions), teaching changes in verbal behavior that can cause the patient's perspective to be more positive, and the use of role-playing to demonstrate the irrationality of certain beliefs (Clark & Martin, 1994).

COGNITIVE-BEHAVIORAL THERAPY FOR TREATMENT OF TINNITUS

Perhaps the most widely used psychological method for treatment of tinnitus is cognitive-behavioral therapy (CBT). J. L. Henry and Wilson (2001) have fully described CBT for treatment of tinnitus and provided specific guidelines for its clinical implementation.

J. L. Henry and Wilson (2001) describe the development of the cognitive-behavioral form of treatment as arising from four principal forms of psychological treatment: (a) hypnosis, (b) biofeedback or relaxation training (also referred to as progressive muscle relaxation training), (c) cognitive restructuring, and (d) attention control/imagery training.

In the late 1980s there was a gradual transition in the thinking of psychological researchers regarding their approach to tinnitus treatment (J. L. Henry & Wilson, 2001). There was decreased emphasis on relaxation training and biofeedback, and increased focus on cognitive aspects of tinnitus. Results of one study (Jakes, Hallam, Rachman, & Hinchcliffe, 1986) showed greater benefit for tinnitus using CBT versus relaxation and biofeedback. Also, numerous non-tinnitus studies have demonstrated the efficacy of CBT for psychological problems (especially depression and anxiety) and for chronic pain. Most importantly, cognitive-behavioral approaches to the treatment of pain were adapted to the management of tinnitus.

The goal of therapy with CBT is to reduce the distress caused by tinnitus (Wilson, 2006). Broad strategies of treatment include (a) cognitive restructuring (modification of maladaptive cognitions), (b) relaxation training, (c) attention control (or attention diversion), and (d) imagery training. The premise of treatment is that the tinnitus has become the focus of attention, and that it is possible for patients to learn to redirect their attention away from their tinnitus using these techniques.

DIRECTIVE COUNSELING FOR TRT

Directive counseling for TRT involves structured educational sessions during which patients are given detailed information designed to create a new frame of reference for thinking about their tinnitus (P. J. Jastreboff & M. M. Jastreboff, 2001). The crucial aspect of the counseling is that it is based strictly on the neurophysiological model of tinnitus (P. J. Jastreboff & Hazell, 2004). Patients are educated about their audiometric test results, auditory structure and function, potential mechanisms of tinnitus generation, and a variety of concepts that relate to the neurophysiological model. The counseling is intended to decrease the strength of neural connections between cortical areas and the limbic and autonomic nervous systems (P. J. Jastreboff & M. M. Jastreboff, 1999). The counseling information should initiate the process of "reclassification" of the tinnitus neural signal that is stored in memory.

During a counseling session, the TRT patient participates in an in-depth discussion in which the source and meaning of the tinnitus are detailed through demonstrations of anatomy, physiology, and examples of various related phenomena to "demystify" the tinnitus. The rationale and importance of maintaining an "enriched" environment of nonannoying sounds to maximize treatment effects are explained. The counseling structure remains essentially the same during each session. However, the nature and detail of the explanations, and the analogies used, depend on the patient's TRT category and will change as patients gain a more educated view of their tinnitus.

A model of the sequential counseling information is provided in the next chapter. Many of the counseling points covered are ideas that audiologists would generally be aware of, such as hair cell function and auditory pathways. Some of the points, however, may be less familiar, such as concepts of consciousness, directed attention, conditioned reflexes, passive extinction, habituation, and the limbic and autonomic nervous systems. These and other specific TRT concepts are explained in the original TRT book (P. J. Jastreboff & Hazell, 2004) and in Part 1 of the present book.

TRT counseling is referred to as directive, and the description provided herein is consistent with that approach. This should not imply, however, that TRT counseling is a strictly one-way process whereby the clinician educates and instructs the patient without regard for the patient's underlying fears and concerns. In fact, it is important to incorporate nondirective components of "Rogerian" counseling to optimize the effectiveness of the counseling. It has been shown in several studies that a more client-centered approach can improve the long-term efficacy of various types of counseling (Stewart et al., 2000). Gagne (1998) offers specific suggestions for applying a client-centered problem-solving approach to audiological rehabilitation, which Gagne considers essential for successful intervention. It is therefore important for the clinician to exhibit an "unconditional positive regard" and an "empathic understanding" toward patients during TRT counseling sessions. By doing so, the patient will realize a greater sense of trust and respect for the clinician, and will feel free to express thoughts and concerns that could otherwise block future progress. It is especially important in TRT counseling that negative and erroneous thoughts and beliefs about tinnitus be dispelled. This, of course, necessitates a warm, interactive relationship between the patient and the clinician. Clark and Martin (1994, p. 60) have articulated well the need for this kind of approach:

> The success or failure of a tinnitus management program, regardless of the procedure used, often turns on the relationship with the patient. Empathy and supportive counseling can be a valuable adjunct to therapeutic intervention. The interpersonal connection that is fostered in such situations may be the factor that determines the efficacy of the program.

13

TRT Counseling

The initial treatment session for TRT consists of the directive counseling protocol, which incorporates fitting of ear-level devices (sound generators or combination instruments) for those patients (Categories 1-4) who require devices as part of their treatment. The counseling protocol is fairly extensive, and it can be difficult for clinicians to present all of the information without referring to some kind of a guide. For this reason the entire counseling protocol is provided in this chapter.

The counseling protocol shown below is presented as a lay-language script (scripted sections in *italics*) that models what clinicians could actually say to their patients. The script demonstrates how the counseling information can be explained in a logical and sequential fashion. (The script, or parts of it, may be read aloud to the patient if necessary.) The scripted counseling is based directly on the description of TRT counseling that has been provided by P. J. Jastreboff and Hazell (2004, Section 3.4, pp. 85-106). In addition, each scripted section corresponds directly to the counseling modules contained in the book (*Tinnitus Retraining Therapy: Patient Counseling Guide*) that was prepared as a companion to the present book. The flip-chart format of the companion book facilitates an orderly counseling session as well as consistency between sessions and between clinicians. With each turn of the page, the clinician is presented with a bulleted list of key counseling points, and the patient is presented with mostly graphics that illustrate the corresponding information. The companion book contains 160 pages of patient counseling materials, including 80 pages oriented to the clinician, and 80 pages for viewing by the patient. (An additional 14 pages are specific to counseling for decreased sound tolerance.) For the initial counseling session, an average of 1 minute or more is required to explain the contents of each page (or module). The entire session can be completed in about 1½ hours, although some patients will require 2 hours or more. In some cases, the counseling should be distributed over two (or more) sessions.

The initial counseling session covers seven major topics: (1) Overview of the auditory system, (2) Hearing and the brain, (3) Rules of perception, (4) Limitation of attention, (5) Plasticity of the brain, (6) The neurophysiological model of tinnitus, and (7) Fitting ear-level devices. (An eighth section is also provided for treatment of decreased sound tolerance in Chapter 15.) For the patient, the session involves a substantial amount of new and fairly technical information that can be difficult to fully comprehend in one sitting. Naturally, patients vary in their ability to learn new information, and the clinician must artfully modify the presentation and improvise accordingly. The main objective is that patients understand the essence of each major concept.

SECTION 1: OVERVIEW OF THE AUDITORY SYSTEM

There are many theories about what causes tinnitus, and no one yet has all the answers. We do, however, know a lot about how the hearing system works. Understanding how we hear can help to "demystify" tinnitus—like opening a "black box" to see what's inside. We're now going to talk about the hearing system, starting with the outer ear and working our way up through the brain. [**Clinician:** An important part of the counseling is explaining to patients the results of their audiological testing. The different test results should be explained where they relate to the different topics in Sections 1 and 2.]

Sound Waves

For every sound that you hear (except your tinnitus), a physical event has taken place somewhere in your "acoustic environment." These physical events create sound waves that emanate from the event in all directions at the same time—like ripples caused by dropping a pebble into a lake (except in three dimensions, like blowing up a balloon). Sound waves transmit energy in an outward direction, and their force causes objects, such as our eardrums, to vibrate.

The Hearing System

*The hearing system can be subdivided into two major divisions: the **ear** and the **auditory nervous system**. The ear is like a microphone (with a built-in amplifier) that collects sound waves and converts them to a different form of energy. The auditory nervous system is analogous to a computer—it processes and interprets the signals coming from the ear. The ear and the auditory nervous system are connected by a "cable"—the **auditory nerve**.*

The Ear

(Figure 13-1) *Most of the ear is encased in bone on the side of the head. The purpose of the ear is to convert sound waves to electrical nerve impulses—like a microphone converts sound waves to electrical impulses. The ear consists of three basic divisions: the outer ear, middle ear, and inner ear.*

*The **outer ear** includes the pinna, which is the part of the ear that can be seen on the side of the head, and the ear canal. The outer ear is the entry point for sound waves that are channeled through the ear canal to the eardrum.*

*The **middle ear** is like a "room" that separates the outer and the inner ears. The purpose of the middle ear is to provide impedance matching between outer and inner ears (which enables the most efficient flow of energy). The eardrum is the outer "wall" of the room. The middle ear bones (malleus, incus, stapes—collectively called the ossicles) are the smallest bones in the body. The ossicles form a "bridge" through which sound waves travel between the eardrum and the inner ear. Tiny muscles connected to the*

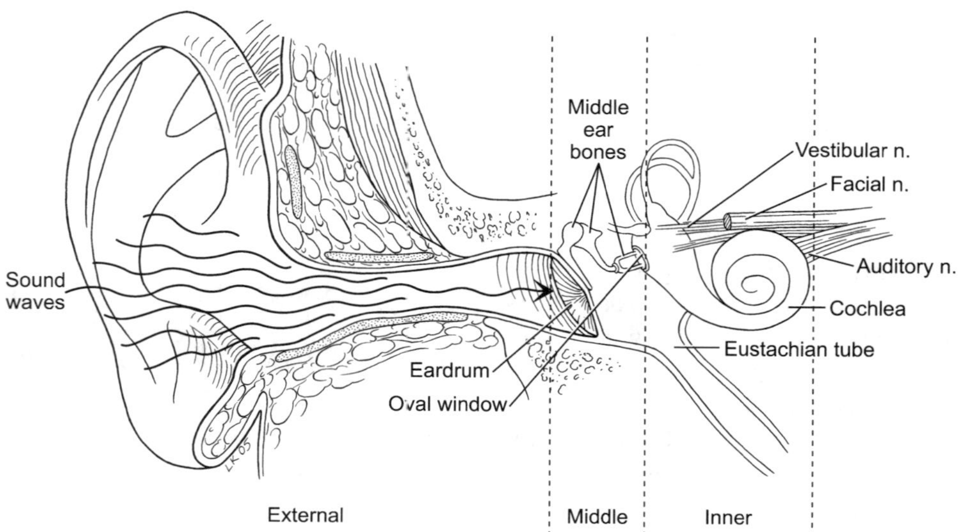

FIGURE 13–1. The ear, showing structures of the outer ear, middle ear, inner ear, and auditory nerve.

ossicles allow the chain to tense up to reduce the intensity of sounds entering the inner ear.

The ***inner ear*** *contains a bony structure called the cochlea, which is shaped like a snail shell and is about the size of a pea. The cochlea is filled with fluid. Sound vibrations from the air must cause movement of the fluid to activate special sensory cells. These sensory cells are called hair cells and they are responsible for converting vibrations to nerve impulses.*

Auditory Nerve: The "Cable"

(Figure 13-1) *The auditory nerve connects the hair cells in the inner ear to the brainstem. This nerve is like a short cable that contains many thousands of wires. Each "wire" in the auditory nerve is an individual nerve fiber.*

Auditory Nervous System: The "Computer"

(Figure 1-4) *Beyond the auditory nerve, there are dedicated areas of the brainstem and brain that process auditory signals. The signals coming from the auditory nerve are relayed through several brain centers as they travel up to the highest level of the brain (the auditory cortex) where "hearing" actually takes place.*

SECTION 2: HEARING AND THE BRAIN

[**Clinician:** This section expands on the previous section by providing much greater detail about how sound waves are converted to nerve impulses and then processed by the brain.] *As a quick summary: Sound waves are received by the ear (the microphone), which converts the vibrations to nerve impulses* (Figure 13-1). *These nerve impulses enter the brain (the computer) by way of the auditory nerve (the cable)* (Figure 1-4). *The impulses undergo processing that becomes increasingly complex as the information travels up through the brain. Hearing is the conscious perception of sound that is coded in these nerve impulses.*

Organ of Corti

(Figure 13-2) *The organ of Corti is the "end-organ of hearing." It is an elaborate structure*

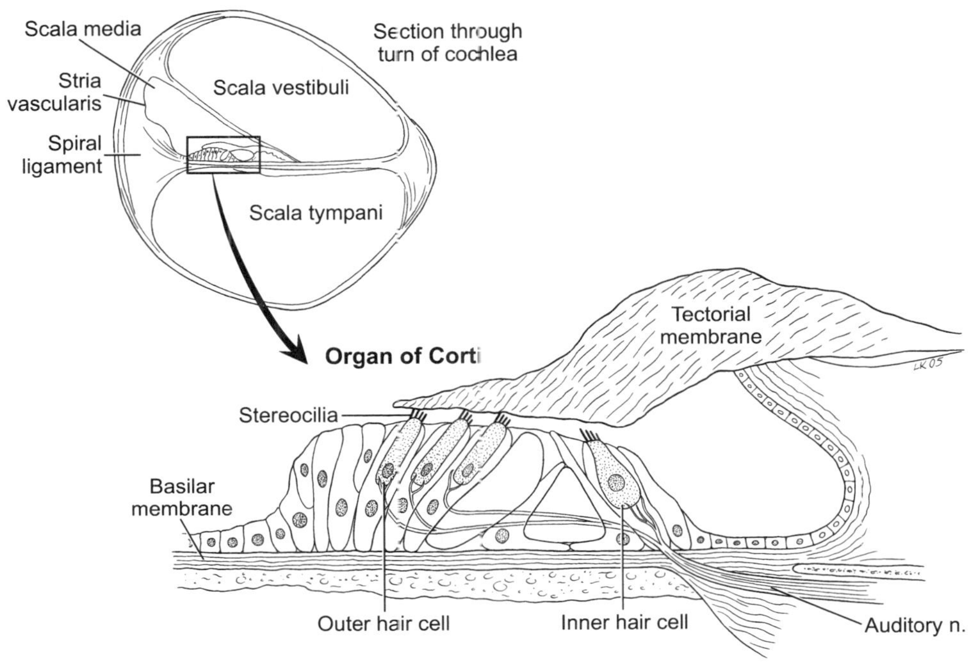

FIGURE 13–2. The organ of Corti.

that is contained within the cochlea. Hair cells that are embedded in the organ of Corti convert vibrations into nerve impulses.

The Piano Keyboard in the Cochlea

(Figure 13–3) *The organ of Corti can be thought of as the "piano keyboard in the cochlea." The hair cells are the "piano keys." On a piano, lower pitches are on the left and higher pitches are on the right. Hair cells are similarly "tuned" from one end of the cochlea to the other—low frequencies at the top and high frequencies at the bottom.*

Hair Cells

(Figures 13–2 and 13–4) *Hair cells are the starting point for auditory neural signals that travel into the brainstem. Each cochlea has about 16,000 hair cells that include inner hair cells and outer hair cells. The cells are distributed evenly along the organ of Corti—one row of inner hair cells next to three rows of outer hair cells.*

The Amplifier in the Cochlea

(Figure 13–2) *Inner hair cells detect sound vibrations and send the information directly into the brain. However, inner hair cells cannot, by themselves, detect vibrations caused by softer sounds. Inner hair cells rely on outer hair cells to mechanically amplify these low-level vibrations to enable their detection.*

Damage to Hair Cells

(Figure 13–5) *Outer hair cells are more susceptible to damage than inner hair cells. Once outer or inner hair cells are destroyed, they cannot recover—at least not in humans. However, temporary damage to hair cells can be caused by loud noise, which usually requires at least a few days for recovery to occur. At some point the damage becomes permanent and the cells cannot recover.*

Loss of Hair Cells and Normal Hearing

(Figure 13–5) *If the outer hair cell loss is diffuse along the organ of Corti, up to 30% of the cells*

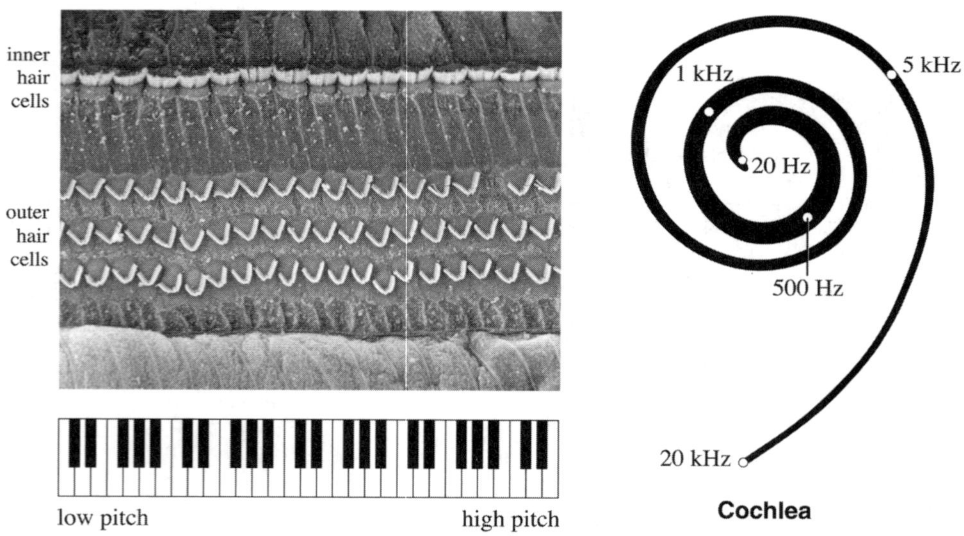

FIGURE 13–3. The hair cells in the organ of Corti (left). There are one row of inner hair cells and three rows of outer hair cells. Shown below is a piano keyboard, representing how the hair cells are laid out with low frequencies on one end progressing to high frequencies on the other. On the right is an artist's rendition of how the different frequencies correspond to different regions of the cochlea. (Photomicrograph courtesy of David J. Lim, MD, House Ear Institute.)

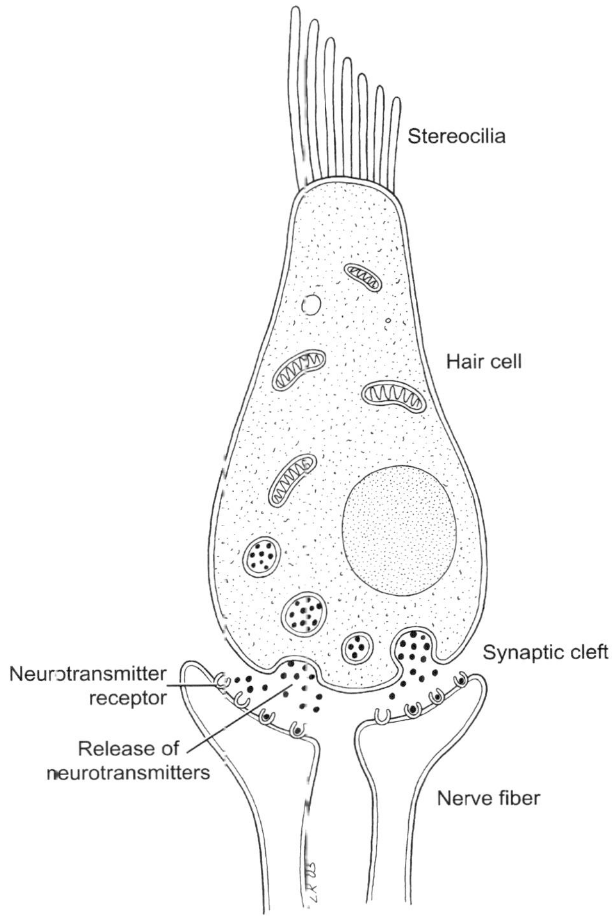

FIGURE 13–4. Schematic representation of an inner hair cell. On the top of the cell are the stereocilia. At the bottom of the cell is the synaptic cleft between the hair cell and the auditory nerve. Signaling between the two takes place by the release of neurotransmitters across the synaptic gap.

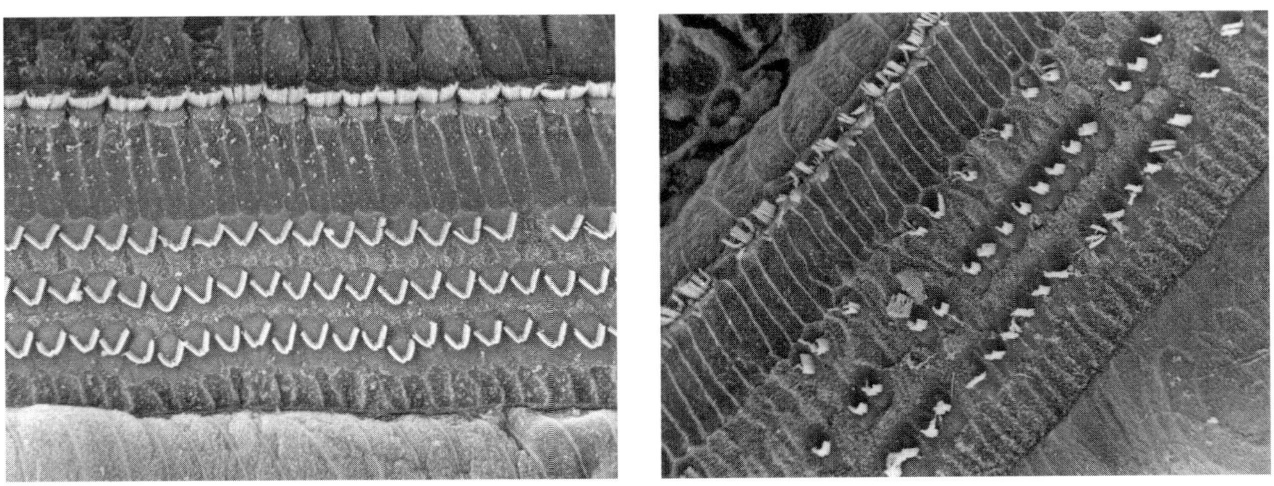

Normal hair cells

Damaged hair cells

FIGURE 13–5. Scanning electron photomicrographs showing surface view of normal chinchilla intact hair cells (left) and a typical pattern of hair cell damage (damaged outer hair cells and intact inner hair cells—right) (1,700 × original magnification). (Photomicrographs courtesy of David J. Lim, MD, House Ear Institute.)

can be lost without affecting the audiogram. This is because hair cells are "redundant"—they can compensate for a certain number of them being lost before the ability to hear is affected. For example, two cells might do the work of three if necessary. We all lose outer hair cells from the moment we are born at the rate of about ½% per year. At that rate, hearing loss would not start to appear until we are around 60 years old. However, there are many factors that can accelerate the damage, such as loud noise, certain ototoxic drugs, viral infections, autoimmune and other medical disorders, and genetic factors. The damage to hair cells tends to start in high frequency regions of the cochlea and progresses to low frequency regions over time.

Hair Cell Loss: Outer versus Inner

(Figure 13–5) *Although there are three times as many outer hair cells as inner hair cells, 95% of the fibers in the auditory nerve come from inner hair cells—only 5% come from outer hair cells. Complete loss of outer hair cells results in about a 50 dB HL flat loss of hearing. Complete loss of inner hair cells—regardless of whether outer hair cells remain—results in total hearing loss. If there is a region in the cochlea with complete loss of inner hair cells, there will be complete loss of hearing in the frequency range that corresponds with that region.*

Otoacoustic Emissions

(Figure 13–5) *Damage to outer hair cells tends to be localized; that is, there are "patches" of damaged cells. Often these patches do not result in any detectable loss of hearing because adjacent healthy cells compensate for the missing cells. These patches, however, may be detectable by distortion-product otoacoustic emissions (DPOAE) testing. Otoacoustic emissions are "echoes" in the ear canal that can be detected only by special equipment. The echoes are caused by the mechanical amplifying action of the outer hair cells. Outer hair cells are literally little muscles that lengthen and shorten in response to vibrations in the cochlear fluid.*

Discordant Damage/Dysfunction

[**Clinician:** Results of the patient's DPOAE testing should be discussed in relation to the audiogram. This is especially important for tinnitus patients who have normal hearing.] (Figure 13–5) *Small areas of damage to outer hair cells may play a role in the emergence of tinnitus. The damage that occurs to outer hair cells results in regions where outer hair cells are damaged and inner hair cells are intact or much less damaged. According to Dr. Jastreboff, these areas of "discordant damage/dysfunction" could be a cause of tinnitus, even when the damage is relatively minor and the hearing is essentially normal* (P. J. Jastreboff, 1990).

Discordant Damage/Dysfunction Theory

(Figure 13–6) *Nerve fibers from the outer and inner hair cells enter the brainstem and synapse in the cochlear nucleus. Fibers from the same region of the cochlea normally balance each other, resulting in normal nerve activity being sent further up the auditory pathways. Specifically, fibers from outer hair cells inhibit the output of fibers from inner hair cells* (Kaltenbach, Zhang, & Zacharek, 2004; Shore, 2004). *When there is discordant damage/dysfunction, fibers from the inner hair cells send their normal excitatory signals, but there are no inhibitory signals coming from the missing outer hair cells. This imbalance is known to cause atypical bursting activity from the dorsal cochlear nucleus* (Kaltenbach et al., 1998). *This bursting activity is amplified by the auditory system and perceived as tinnitus.*

Neural Networks

(Figure 1–2) *Neural pathways lead from the cochlea all the way to the cortex. These pathways are very complex, and consist of series of interconnected nerve cells, called neural networks, that process the auditory signals. Auditory processing includes recognition of neural patterns and blocking of signals that are unimportant or not relevant to the current activity.*

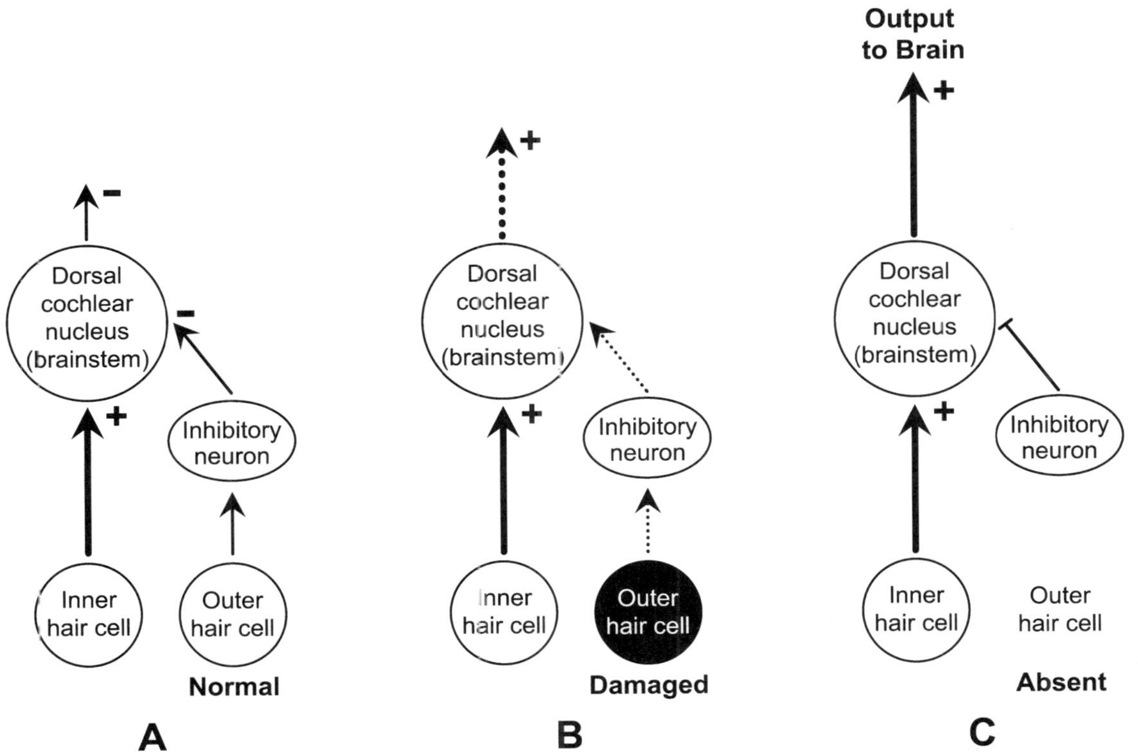

FIGURE 13–6. Schematic representation of discordant damage/dysfunction theory. **A.** Normal transmission of signals from undamaged inner and outer hair cells. The outer hair cells (OHCs) exert an inhibitory effect on the dorsal cochlear nucleus (DCN) via inhibitory neurons. The arrow coming from the top of the DCN (labeled with a negative sign) is the output to the brain, and it is proportionally shorter than the outputs shown in B and C to indicate that the output from the DCN is normally inhibited by OHCs. **B.** Output from the DCN is greater than in A because inhibitory OHC input to the DCN is reduced due to OHC damage/dysfunction. **C.** Output from the DCN is greater than in B because OHCs are absent; thus, all OHC inhibition on the DCN is lost. The result is a completely uninhibited output signal to the brain. Either scenario in B or C represents enhanced auditory activity due to discordant damage/dysfunction between inner and outer hair cells. (Figure modified from *Tinnitus Retraining Therapy: Implementing the Neurophysiological Model* (Figure 2.5, p. 28), by P. J. Jastreboff & J. W. P. Hazell, 2004, New York: Cambridge University Press. Adapted with permission.)

Enhancement and Suppression of Neural Activity

(Figure 13–7) *Connections between individual neurons have two basic features: (a) They can cause either enhancement or suppression of activity and (b) they continually undergo change. As changes occur in these connections, the "sending" neuron's impact on the "receiving" neuron can either increase or decrease. Networks of neurons (neural networks) can process many different signals at the same time* (Figure 1–2). *Some of these signals will be enhanced and some will be suppressed.*

Auditory Gain

The auditory system has a "gain control," like the volume control on a stereo. The level of gain determines the degree to which environmental sounds are amplified, or enhanced. The level of

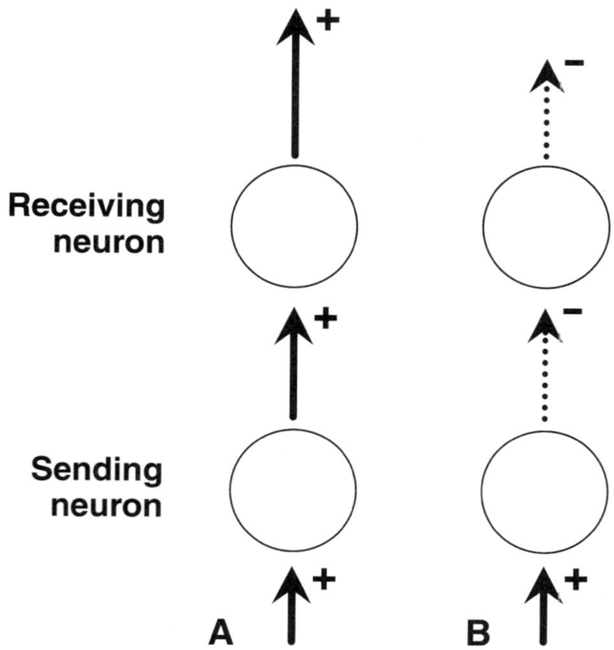

FIGURE 13–7. Schematic representation of enhancement and suppression of neural activity. Both A and B show series transmission of activity between successive neurons. The "sending" neuron is at the bottom and the "receiving" neuron is at the top. **A.** The sending neuron is exerting excitatory activity onto the receiving neuron, resulting in enhanced output from the receiving neuron. **B.** The sending neuron is exerting inhibitory activity onto the receiving neuron, resulting in reduced output from the receiving neuron.

gain changes automatically to adjust to the level of sound. As the sound level decreases, the gain increases. As the sound level increases, the gain decreases. This gain is controlled partially by the outer hair cells, which mechanically amplify sounds, and partially by neural networks that respond to different levels of sound.

The Heller and Bergman Experiment

This experiment was performed over 50 years ago but is very significant for all tinnitus patients (Heller & Bergman, 1953). *In the experiment, individuals without tinnitus were placed in a sound booth and asked to write down "any sounds they might hear." Within 5 minutes of sitting in the sound booth, 94% of the 80 individuals who were tested reported buzzing, pulsing, and whistling sounds identical to sounds reported by tinnitus sufferers. This experiment demonstrated that the perception of tinnitus is an inherent property of the auditory nervous system under certain circumstances. Thus, tinnitus is not necessarily the result of a pathological process.*

Why Is the Heller and Bergman Experiment Important?

Individual nerve fibers in the auditory nervous system discharge spontaneously 50–100 times each second. This is random activity that occurs when there is no sound. When sound occurs, the random activity becomes more patterned. The brain recognizes different patterns of activity as different sounds. The patterned activity travels through the auditory nerve and up the auditory pathways, finally reaching the auditory cortex where sound is perceived (see Figure 1–4). *The processing that occurs allows the patterned activity to be recognized as sound. At the same time, the background random activity is filtered out and is not perceived as sound. If there is a decrease in auditory activity, however, auditory gain increases. Thus, when a person's acoustic environment is sufficiently quiet (for example, in a sound booth), the brain may detect fluctuations in the spontaneous activity that are interpreted as sound—hence, tinnitus. According to the Heller and Bergman experiment, almost everyone has tinnitus if it is quiet enough. For many people, therefore, tinnitus may be a side effect of a normal compensatory mechanism to minor changes in the cochlea.*

SECTION 3: RULES OF PERCEPTION

When you have your hearing tested, the objective is to identify the softest sounds that you can detect in a quiet environment. In real life, however, hearing normally involves the detection of complex sounds in the presence of other complex sounds. We can recognize individual sounds because our neural networks have been trained, through repeated exposure to the sounds, to recognize the patterns of neural activity that are associated with the sounds. When a certain sound has special meaning, such as our name, our auditory system becomes "tuned" to detect the sound. That is why we notice our name being mentioned in a noisy environment, even when we are engaged in a separate conversation. (This is known as the "cocktail party effect.") This tuning effect can also happen with tinnitus. Its continuous presence can train neural networks to detect the signal with high precision. If importance is attached to the tinnitus signal, the signal will be easily detectable by the brain even in the presence of other auditory signals.

Perception of Signal Strength

When we are exposed to any kind of stimulus, or "signal," one of the qualities of the signal that we perceive is its "strength." This perception of signal strength is not based only on the absolute physical intensity of the signal. The perception of signal strength depends mostly upon the ***relative*** *strength of the signal compared to other surrounding signals. For example, a burning candle in a dark room appears very bright and cannot be ignored* (Figure 13–8). *The same candle in a brightly lit room, however, is barely noticeable. As another example, while driving we adjust the car radio to be loud enough to be heard comfortably over the road noise. When we park and shut off the engine, the radio suddenly seems too loud. The radio did not get louder—it is just perceived as louder because of the elimination of background noise.*

Perception of Tinnitus Strength

(Figure 13–9) *Just like a car radio seems to become louder when the car is parked and the engine is turned off, our tinnitus seems to get louder when we climb into bed after a busy day. When we finally lie down, all of the background sound suddenly stops. It is this silence that causes our tinnitus to seem to be louder. This points out why it is so important to* ***avoid silence****. We should always maintain some background sound to reduce the* ***perception*** *of the loudness of the tinnitus, and to decrease the strength of the tinnitus neural signal.*

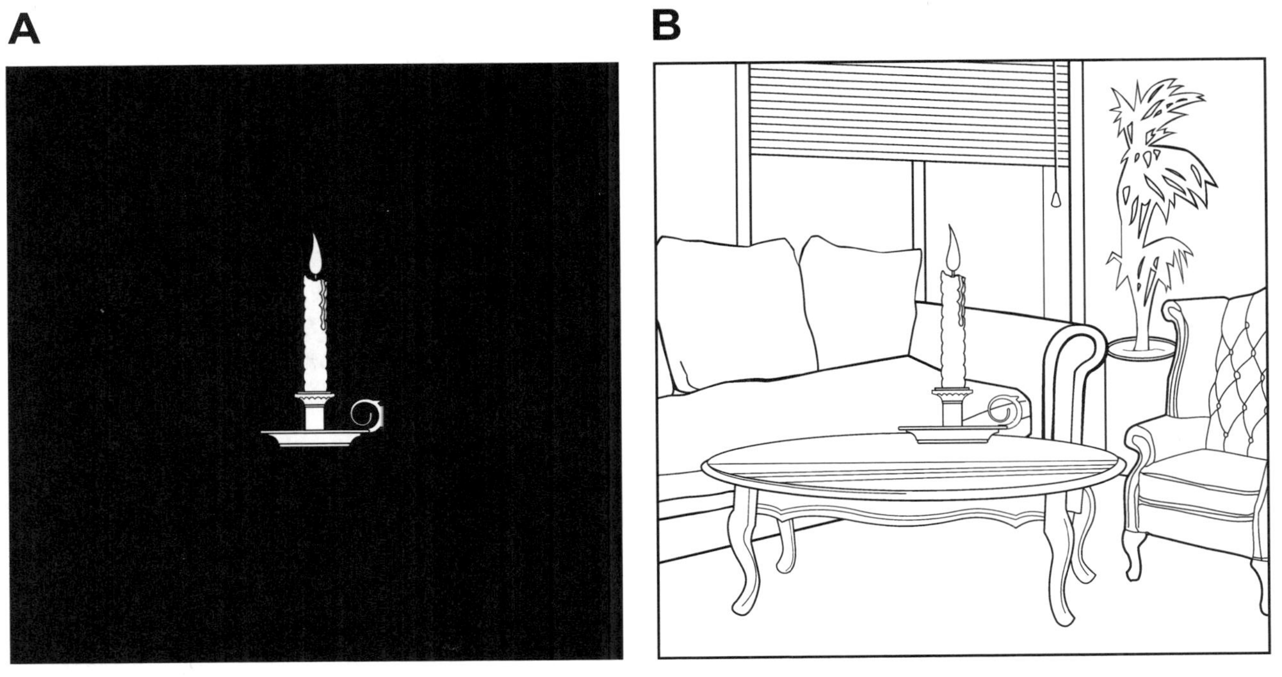

FIGURE 13–8. A. Candle in a dark room. **B.** Candle in a lighted room. The candle is the same in both figures, but is less noticeable in the lighted room because of the reduced contrast.

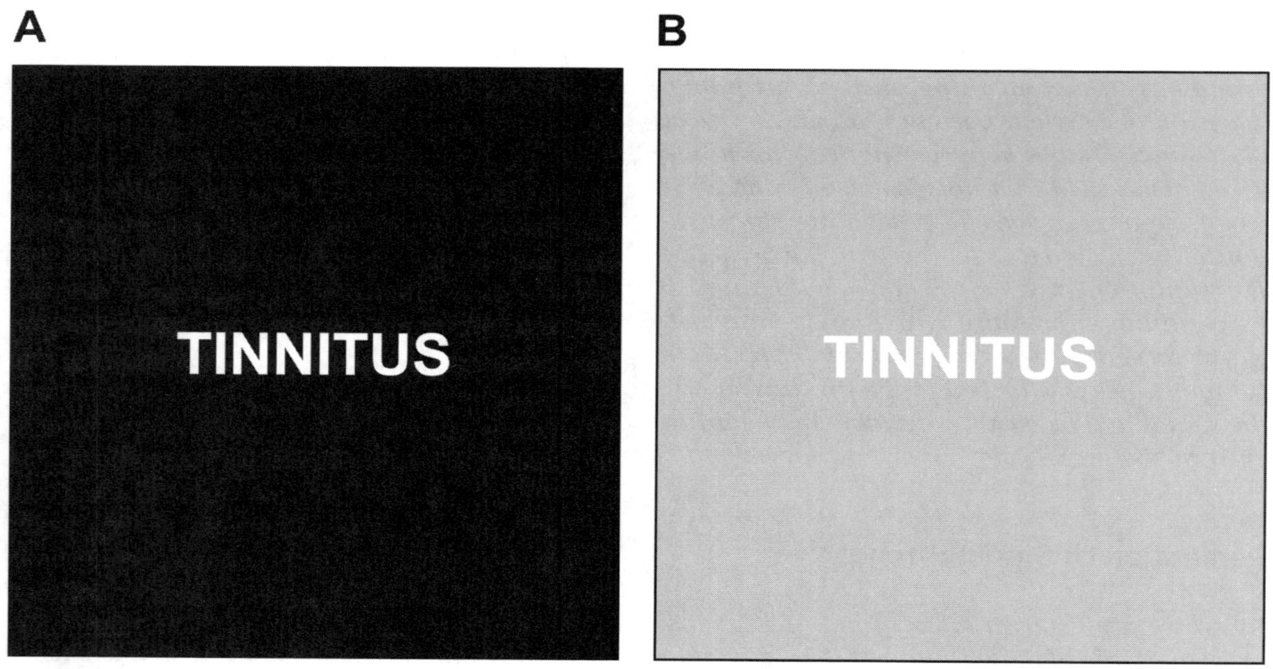

FIGURE 13–9. As for the candle in Figure 13–8, the word "tinnitus" is the same in both A and B, but is less noticeable in B because of the reduced contrast.

SECTION 4: LIMITATION OF ATTENTION

Although the brain can perform many complex tasks, it can only perform one complex conscious task requiring our attention at a time. Two examples of complex tasks are reading a book and writing a letter. We cannot do both of these at the same time.

Sensory Overload

Our senses are usually flooded with information. Our auditory system alone must process numerous sounds, most of which do not get our attention. All of the sounds activate the inner ear, which converts the vibrations to neural signals that are sent into the brain for processing. The brain uses several strategies to distinguish and separate the many signals so that only those that are most relevant to our current task reach our awareness. We are going to discuss three of those strategies.

Managing Sensory Overload: (1) Automated Responses

Many tasks do not require our conscious attention—they are almost automatic. These kinds of tasks can be accomplished because of ***conditioned reflexes****. For example, walking, running, climbing stairs, or riding a bike—each of these tasks involves routine, predictable responses. Playing a musical instrument becomes almost automatic with practice. Even driving a car, which requires continuous processing of a huge amount of complex information, can be done while carrying on a conversation.*

Managing Sensory Overload: (2) Classification of Signals

All sensory information that enters the brain is classified into two categories: (a) important and (b) unimportant. If a signal is classified as important, that means the brain has learned that there is some consequence to the signal. In other words, the signal has resulted in ***rein-***

forcement—*either reward or punishment. Whenever an important stimulus is experienced, it will not be blocked from reaching conscious attention. An important signal will typically require some action to be taken (at least paying attention to the signal). In contrast, a stimulus becomes classified as unimportant if it is experienced repeatedly with no reinforcement. Such a "neutral" stimulus will not evoke a reaction, and it may not even be noticed.*

Managing Sensory Overload: (3) Prioritization of Signals

Signals also are ***ranked according to their relative importance****. Signals requiring immediate attention are dealt with first, and others are dealt with in order of decreasing priority. Signals that induce fear or are perceived as threatening cause immediate action. If we are out in the woods, the sound of an approaching tiger will dominate our attention until we are (hopefully) out of danger. This is an automatic response over which we have no control. Similarly, if there is a tiger lying in the corner during a counseling session, the tiger will completely draw attention away from the conversation—even with assurance that the tiger is friendly. If tinnitus is perceived as threatening in any way, it can cause the same type of reaction.*

SECTION 5: PLASTICITY OF THE BRAIN

A basic characteristic of the brain is that it undergoes continuous change—the brain is "plastic." These changes occur in the connections between neurons (synapses), including new connections and modifications in the strength of existing connections (Figure 13-4). *These connections are the basis for acquiring new memories, both for conscious information and for conditioned reflexes. It is a common observation that having to* ***relearn*** *something takes longer than if nothing was learned initially. We can learn to perfect our golf swing, but if the swing is already incorrect the learning will take longer than if we had never swung a golf club.*

Retraining of Conditioned Reflexes

Conditioned reflexes, once learned, can be relearned (or retrained). The retraining process, however, requires the performance of certain exercises over a period of time. Retraining cannot occur through a strictly cognitive process. When tinnitus becomes a problem, the auditory neural signal for the tinnitus has become linked to parts of the brain that are responsible for feelings of annoyance and stress. This link is a conditioned reflex, which must be "extinguished" through proper exercises. Since a strong emotional association has been learned, the relearning process normally requires a period of months to as long as a year or more.

Nonauditory Systems Activated by Tinnitus

There are different systems within the brain. Each system has a specific function, but there is also interaction between systems. The auditory nervous system processes auditory information. Tinnitus is a signal in the auditory nervous system, and this signal can affect other systems. The kinds of problems caused by tinnitus indicate that the ***limbic system*** *and the* ***autonomic nervous system*** *can become activated by the tinnitus signal.*

Limbic System

(Figure 4-1) *The limbic system is the part of the brain that is responsible for emotions. There are direct connections between the limbic system and the auditory nervous system. It is through these connections that sounds can evoke emotional responses due to their association with certain memories. Music, a crying baby, or a particular person's voice can cause emotional reactions.* ***If a sound does not cause activity in the limbic system, the sound will be spontaneously and automatically habituated.***

Autonomic Nervous System

(Figure 5-1) *The autonomic nervous system controls basic bodily functions such as heartbeat, blood pressure, breathing, body temperature, sweating, and so on. These are automatic functions that we cannot normally control. To an extent, these functions can be modified by exercising or relaxing. Also, techniques such as biofeedback and hypnosis can provide a certain amount of control over the autonomic nervous system.*

Fight-or-Flight Response

(Figure 5-1) *The autonomic nervous system becomes strongly activated when there is danger or fear. Specifically, the* ***sympathetic*** *part of the autonomic nervous system induces changes in the body that prepare it for* ***fight-or-flight****. These changes include release of adrenaline into the bloodstream, increased muscle tension, increased heart rate, increased rate of respiration, and shutting down of digestive processes. The fight-or-flight reaction is so powerful that it can be sustained for only a brief period of time.*

Chronic Stress

(Figure 5-1) *The autonomic nervous system also is activated when there is no fear or danger. Whenever the body is presented with the need for either a physical or mental action, the sympathetic part of the autonomic nervous system is activated. This is a normal response, but it can become abnormal if the activation is* ***sustained****. Thus, a person does not need to have the fight-or-flight reaction to have a problem with overactivation of the autonomic nervous system, which is referred to as* ***chronic stress****. The level and duration of the activation determine whether the effects cause unhealthy consequences. Chronic stress can result in sleep deprivation, exhaustion, and many other deleterious effects on health. These effects reduce or prevent the ability to experience normal quality-of-life activities.*

Tinnitus and Stress

If the tinnitus signal acquires negative associations, the continual monitoring of the signal (both consciously and subconsciously) can cause constant activation of the sympathetic part of the autonomic nervous system. The level of sustained activation depends on the severity of the tinnitus and the strength of the negative associations.

SECTION 6: THE NEUROPHYSIOLOGICAL MODEL OF TINNITUS

To review briefly, we have discussed the auditory nervous system, limbic system, and autonomic nervous system. The auditory nervous system processes neural signals so that we can hear and understand sounds. Some sounds evoke an emotional reaction, which is caused by activation of the limbic system (Figure 4-1). *Activation of the limbic system by a stimulus that has negative associations causes activity in the sympathetic part of the autonomic nervous system* (Figure 5-1). *(In contrast, if the stimulus has positive associations—for example, pleasant music—the* ***parasympathetic*** *part of the autonomic nervous system is activated. Parasympathetic activation counteracts sympathetic activation.) If the sympathetic activity is extreme, profound changes in the body will occur that prepare it for flight-or-flight. If the activity is less than extreme, but sustained for a long period of time, the same reactions will occur but to a lesser degree. Again, these reactions can be caused by any activation of the sympathetic nervous system—not just fight-or-flight.*

Conditioned Reflexes

(Figure 4-2) *It is important to understand that the tinnitus signal all by itself is harmless. The signal becomes a problem only when it becomes linked to the limbic and autonomic nervous systems, which are governed by conditioned reflexes. Conditioned reflexes caused by tinnitus are inappropriate because they cause the body to react to a harmless stimulus. This can happen to different degrees. As the autonomic nervous system becomes more activated, the corresponding perception is that the severity of the tinnitus has increased.*

No-Problem Tinnitus

(Figure 4-2) *For about 80% of all people who experience tinnitus, the tinnitus does not acquire any special meaning, and a natural process of "spontaneous habituation" takes place. The tinnitus is thus classified by the brain as an* ***unimportant*** *signal. The brain learns that the tinnitus signal is insignificant, like the sound of a new refrigerator, and the signal is normally blocked from activating the limbic and autonomic nervous systems, and from reaching consciousness—the tinnitus signal is there but the person is not normally aware of it.*

Problem Tinnitus

(Figure 4-2) *For the other 20% of people with tinnitus, it's a different story. For these people, their tinnitus* ***does*** *acquire special meaning because of its association with something negative (the signal is classified as* ***important****). This association normally takes place when the tinnitus is first experienced—because an unpleasant or traumatic event takes place at the same time. The anxiety and annoyance caused by the event become linked to the tinnitus. From the perspective of the neurophysiological model, an active connection is established between the auditory nervous system, where the tinnitus signal originates, and the limbic and autonomic nervous systems. This connection increases the activity in the limbic and autonomic nervous systems, which is what causes tinnitus to be a clinically significant condition. When this occurs, the patient pays more attention to the tinnitus, which only worsens the condition.*

The Vicious Circle

(Figure 4-2) *When tinnitus is first experienced, it is only natural to be concerned about this new and intrusive sound. The initial concerns may escalate into feelings of annoyance and anxiety, which are manifestations of an activated limbic system. When this occurs, the tinnitus signal takes on the meaning of a threatening stimulus. Any auditory signal that is recognized as threatening will receive special attention by certain neural networks that become highly tuned to monitor the signal. The tinnitus signal is processed like any other auditory signal in this regard. An increase in detection of the tinnitus signal leads to further activation of the limbic and autonomic nervous systems, which, in turn, further enhances detection. A vicious circle is thus established between the perception of tinnitus and the annoyance caused by tinnitus.*

Effects of Tinnitus

(Figure 4-2) *The vicious circle just described results in a high level of activation of the sympathetic part of the autonomic nervous system (stress response). This activation can cause many effects on the body, including heart fluctuations, digestive problems, and nausea. Some patients experience enhanced perception affecting all of the senses—referred to as "global hypersensitivity." Most patients experience an enhanced perception of their tinnitus during sleep due to the quiet environment. Although tinnitus can interfere with falling asleep, it is more often reported to interfere with maintaining sleep.*

Sleep Deprivation

If tinnitus interferes with sleep on a nightly basis, sleep deprivation can add to any effects already caused by the tinnitus. It may be difficult to distinguish between effects caused by the tinnitus and those caused by the sleep deprivation. These effects include exhaustion, irritability, illogical thinking, perceptual distortions, and difficulty in performing tasks that require prolonged concentration (Carlson, 1991). *There also may be a tendency to make irrational associations, which can lead to further annoyance due to the tinnitus.*

Medications for Sleep

Many tinnitus patients use medications to help them sleep. These drugs may increase the length of sleep, but they also may suppress REM (rapid eye movement) sleep, which is an essential sleep stage that normally occurs four to five times a night. Some of these drugs also directly affect the limbic system, which may be the only way to relieve severe distress due to tinnitus. Such use of drugs may be necessary for a short period, but their long-term use will not break the vicious circle of tinnitus reaction and perception. Drugs may also produce negative side effects, as well as dependence on their use. Moreover, the use of drugs can actually cause tinnitus or exacerbate existing tinnitus.

Tinnitus Loudness and Tinnitus Severity

A tinnitus evaluation usually includes an assessment of the loudness and pitch of the tinnitus. It has been a common observation that these measurements are not related to the suffering caused by the tinnitus. For example, a measurement may show that the person's tinnitus is not loud, but the person may be very distressed by the tinnitus. Or a measurement may indicate that the tinnitus is very loud, yet the person is not bothered by it. The measurement of the tinnitus, which reflects activity in the auditory nervous system, is thus irrelevant to the severity of the tinnitus. What affects the severity is the level of activation of the autonomic nervous system. This is a very important point to understand.

Autonomic Nervous System Activity

The autonomic nervous system has different levels of activity. Low levels of activity in the sympathetic part of the autonomic nervous system reflect a relaxed state, while high levels are associated with stress. The highest level is the fight-or-flight condition. The level of autonomic activity at the time the tinnitus is first experienced can influence the degree to which the tinnitus becomes a problem. If the preexisting autonomic nervous system activity is low, then the likelihood is to naturally habituate to the tinnitus. If the preexisting activity is high, then the tinnitus can further increase the activity—leading to the vicious circle. This may explain why tinnitus that emerges during a period of high stress can become such a severe problem (Hazell, 1996a).

Conscious Loop

(Figure 4–2) *There are essentially two systems in the brain that control activity in the limbic and autonomic nervous systems. One is a system that is dominated by conscious thought processes (the "conscious loop"), while the other is dominated by subconscious processes (the "subconscious loop"). The conscious loop involves interconnections between the cortex and the limbic system. Conscious thoughts that are related to the tinnitus can be greatly affected by fears that are associated with the tinnitus. A person can have fears that the tinnitus means there is a brain tumor, impending deafness, or a mental disorder. Having these kinds of thoughts can directly affect the activity of the autonomic nervous system.*

Subconscious Loop

(Figure 4–2) *The subconscious loop involves interconnections between the limbic and autonomic nervous systems. This loop does not involve conscious thoughts, but it can have the same, if not larger, effects on the limbic and autonomic nervous systems. The subconscious loop is generally caused by the establishment of conditioned reflexes, and can result in chronic annoyance or anxiety. There also can be sleep disruption and problems with concentration. Some patients even experience panic attacks that seem to occur spontaneously. All of these effects can take place without any awareness of the tinnitus. For most patients, both conscious and subconscious loops are active in causing the mental, emotional, and sleep problems that are associated with tinnitus. For all patients who are bothered by their tinnitus, however, the subconscious loop is at least partially involved.*

Reacting Constantly to Tinnitus

(Figure 4-2) *With regard to tinnitus, the subconscious loop may be more important than the conscious loop. The subconscious loop involves learned, or conditioned, responses that occur automatically. The fact that tinnitus is always present can mean that there is a constant subconscious reaction to the tinnitus. This constancy of tinnitus can make it much more difficult to treat than if it only occurred occasionally.*

Experiencing a New Sound

(Figure 4-2) *When a new sound is first experienced, it activates the auditory pathways up to the cortex. Because the sound is new, it receives attention by the auditory system and is evaluated in the cortex to determine its meaning. At the same time, the new signal evokes mild activity in the limbic and autonomic nervous systems.*

Natural Habituation to a New Sound

(Figure 4-2) *If no responsive action is required to a new sound, the signal will be classified as "unimportant." Further exposure to the sound will result in a weakening of the reactive activity in the limbic and autonomic nervous systems. The sound will still undergo detection by the auditory system, but it will not stimulate the limbic and autonomic nervous systems. This describes the process of habituation to a meaningless signal—the signal is detected, but it does not reach conscious perception.*

New Refrigerator

A new refrigerator provides a good example of natural habituation. When first installed, the refrigerator's sound is new and it gets our attention. The sound may seem intrusive, which could cause some slight annoyance and mild activation of the autonomic nervous system. We may even think that the sound indicates malfunction, which can cause anxiety and further activation of the autonomic nervous system. A check with the dealer may provide reassurance that the refrigerator is functioning normally. The information provided by the dealer addresses our concerns, and there is no reason to continue to monitor the refrigerator's sound—it is still there but we do not pay attention to it.

Classification of New Sound: "Important"

(Figure 4-2) *Any new sound is classified by the brain as "high priority" relative to other sounds in the environment. With any new sound, there is initially a perception of the sound and some **mild** reaction. The sound must be evaluated to determine (a) if the sound is important or unimportant, (b) if the sound indicates danger, and (c) if any action is needed.*

Reclassification of New Sound: "Unimportant"

*For sounds such as a new refrigerator, we learn that the sound is meaningless, and subsequently the signal becomes classified by the brain as "unimportant." Because of this classification, we now no longer perceive the sound most of the time, and the sound does not cause any annoyance when it is perceived. What has taken place in the brain? The "unimportant" classification has caused the signal to be "filtered" at subconscious levels. The signal no longer maintains a connection with the limbic and autonomic nervous systems—indicating that the **reactions** to the sound have habituated. Such a filtered signal also does not normally activate pathways leading to the auditory cortex, which indicates that habituation of the **perception** of the sound has taken place.*

New Tinnitus

When tinnitus is first experienced, it undergoes the same evaluation process as for any other new sound. Some patients think that the new tinnitus sound is coming from somewhere in the environment, and they may search for the source of the sound. In some cases, they are convinced that there is a sound, which may lead to an analysis of sounds in the environment. A particular group of patients, referred to as "hummers," think that they hear low-frequency sounds that seem to come from electrical transformers or gas pipes (Rice, 1994). *Most people with tinnitus of recent onset realize quickly that their tinnitus perception does not change as they move around the environment and as they move in and out of different environments. They realize that the sound originates within the head.*

Habituation Occurs above the Tinnitus Generator

(Figure 4–2) *The **cure** for tinnitus would be to eliminate it at its source. This cannot be done presently, although research is ongoing with the objective of finding a way to consistently reduce its perception. Nevertheless, as we have discussed, it is not the perception of tinnitus but rather the reactions to it that cause the problems. Fortunately, it is possible to habituate both the reactions to the tinnitus and the perception of the tinnitus. Just like water extinguishes a fire, there are special techniques that are designed to "extinguish" the conditioned reflexes that occur in association with the tinnitus. The habituation process takes place above the source of the tinnitus in the auditory nervous system; thus, even though the tinnitus signal itself is unaffected, the reactions are stopped. This helps to explain why measurements of tinnitus loudness and pitch are not relevant to the degree of suffering caused by the tinnitus. It also means that the cause of the tinnitus is irrelevant—habituation can occur regardless of the cause or the diagnosis of tinnitus.*

Main Goal of Treatment with TRT

(Figure 4–2) *The main goal of treatment with TRT is habituation of the **reactions** to tinnitus. When this occurs, the person no longer exhibits clinically significant negative reactions to the tinnitus despite the fact that the audiologically measured loudness and pitch of the tinnitus may remain unchanged. The percentage of time the person is aware of the tinnitus may also stay the same. In essence, the tinnitus stops impacting the person's life even though there is still awareness of the tinnitus. This goal can be accomplished only by changing the functional connections between the tinnitus signal in the auditory system and its activation of the limbic and autonomic nervous systems. These connections are responsible for the conditioned reflex arc that ultimately activates the sympathetic part of the autonomic nervous system. Note that once at least partial habituation of reaction is achieved, the subjective perception of tinnitus loudness decreases due to lack of input to the auditory system from the limbic and autonomic nervous systems.*

Secondary Goal of Treatment with TRT

(Figure 4–2) *The secondary goal of treatment with TRT is habituation of the **perception** of tinnitus. When this is accomplished, the person is unaware of the tinnitus most of the time. The tinnitus is still there—meaning the tinnitus signal is still active in the auditory nervous system. However, the signal is normally blocked from reaching consciousness. That is, the signal does not reach the level in the brain (the cortex) where it is perceived. Habituation of perception occurs automatically once a sufficient level of habituation of reactions is achieved.*

Habituation and Passive Extinction

*Habituation and passive extinction refer to essentially the same learning process. The first goal of TRT is **habituation of the reactions to tinnitus**, which is also referred to as **passive***

extinction of conditioned reflexes. *Passive extinction of conditioned reflexes was first described by Pavlov* (Konorski, 1948). *Understanding these concepts about learning is crucial to understanding how tinnitus habituation occurs.*

Passive Extinction of Conditioned Reflexes

(Figure 4-2) *The neurophysiological model shows how the auditory nervous system is connected to the autonomic nervous system. These connections have a subconscious loop and a conscious loop. The connections cannot be modified directly, so we rely on a specific method of passive extinction of conditioned reflexes. A stimulus acquires meaning because it becomes associated with some reinforcement. If the stimulus is presented repeatedly without the reinforcement, then passive extinction of the conditioned (or learned) reflexes will take place. The learning that takes place is that the stimulus is no longer associated with the reinforcement. With tinnitus, the stimulus is the tinnitus signal, and the (negative) reinforcement is the reactions of the autonomic nervous system. For the tinnitus patient it is not possible to eliminate all reactions to the tinnitus; thus, the classic method of passive extinction must be used in a modified fashion. For TRT, the method is modified by* ***reducing*** *(not eliminating) the negative reinforcement, while at the same time the strength of the tinnitus signal is decreased by sound therapy (described later).*

Reclassification of Tinnitus

(Figure 4-2) *For passive extinction to work with tinnitus, we must reduce the reactions that occur in the autonomic nervous system in response to the tinnitus signal. There are four ways that this is accomplished.* ***First****, at the conscious level the tinnitus signal must be reclassified as an unimportant (or "neutral") stimulus. We've discussed how tinnitus occurs as a side effect of normal compensation in the auditory nervous system. This compensation can take place because of damaged outer hair cells (the discordant damage/dysfunction theory of tinnitus generation), or because of an extremely quiet environment that causes enhancement of gain within the auditory nervous system (recall the Heller and Bergman experiment). When the tinnitus becomes reclassified as a neutral signal at the cognitive (thinking) level of the brain, then the conscious loop affecting autonomic nervous system activity is either broken, or the connections are strongly reduced. When this reclassification is achieved, only the subconscious loop continues to activate the autonomic nervous system. Reclassification of tinnitus to a neutral signal must occur in order for habituation to take place.*

Known Danger versus Unknown Danger

The ***second*** *way to reduce autonomic reactions makes use of the psychological principle that* ***known*** *danger causes weaker reactions in the autonomic nervous system than* ***unknown*** *danger. For example, a dental patient who requires a procedure will be less anxious about the procedure if there has been a clear explanation of what is involved—compared to no explanation. With respect to tinnitus, we make use of this principle by explaining possible mechanisms of tinnitus perception and why tinnitus causes negative emotional reactions. The neurophysiological model provides the framework for explaining these concepts. Understanding these concepts can in turn reduce the activity in the autonomic nervous system that is caused by the tinnitus.*

Thinking Positively about Tinnitus

The ***third*** *way to reduce autonomic reactions is to create new associations with the tinnitus that are positive. We try not to think about the sound of tinnitus in negative terms, but in positive terms, such as, "Tinnitus is the music of the brain." This treatment is all about achieving success, and there is good reason to believe that* *success is likely. Many clinical reports have consistently demonstrated successful results with TRT* (P. J. Jastreboff & Hazell, 2004). *Recently, research has shown that TRT is effective for most patients, and even more effective for patients with the greatest tinnitus severity* (Figure 13–10) (J. A. Henry, Schechter, et al., 2005; J. A. Henry et al., 2006a, 2006b). *There is good reason to be hopeful about a successful outcome of treatment. Positive thoughts and feelings of hope will result in reduced activity in the autonomic nervous system.*

Stress Management

*A **fourth** way to reduce activity in the autonomic nervous system is to reduce the overall level of stress. Most tinnitus patients live lives that are very stressful, both at work and at home, and these stresses all contribute to the overall level of activity in the autonomic nervous system. It is therefore helpful to use various methods of stress management. More formal methods of stress management include relaxation training, biofeedback, and hypnosis. Less formally, good time management and a variety of recreational activities can reduce stress. Any of these methods can help to weaken feedback loops that are responsible for maintaining a high level of annoyance in response to the tinnitus signal. Importantly, however, even good stress management is not generally sufficient to achieve permanent habituation to tinnitus.*

Distraction Techniques

Methods of distraction are often used to get relief from annoying tinnitus. These strategies can be helpful on a short-term basis, but in the long run they are counterproductive with respect to long-term habituation to tinnitus. Distraction from tinnitus works only when the person is actively thinking about the tinnitus. Distraction does not have any effect on the connection between the auditory nervous system and the limbic system. Thus, if that connection is causing activity in the autonomic nervous system, distraction will cause no change in the connection, and habituation of the reactions to tinnitus will not occur. Distraction techniques can even have the opposite effect of attracting attention to the tinnitus.

Sound Therapy

*We have discussed how to achieve passive extinction of conditioned reflexes to tinnitus through the use of various techniques. None of these techniques has involved the therapeutic use of sound. We will now discuss the use of **sound therapy** to facilitate extinction of conditioned reflexes. Counseling and sound therapy are the two indispensable components of TRT. The overall purpose of sound therapy in this regard is to **decrease the strength of the tinnitus signal**. This is accomplished through the use of sound, and does not necessitate the use of any particular device. It is important when using any kind of device for sound therapy that the device produces a high quality of sound and that the sound is comfortable and nonannoying.*

Reducing Contrast = Reducing Strength

(Figures 4–2, 13–8, 13–9) *Our perception of the strength of a stimulus is based on the contrast between the stimulus and the background. This is often referred to as the figure-ground relationship. For example, written words are most detectable when they appear in black against a white background. A burning candle in a dark room seems brighter than the same candle when the lights are on. Likewise, the strength of the tinnitus neural signal depends on the background neural activity. As the background neural activity is increased, the strength of the tinnitus neural signal is perceived as weaker within the brain. Sound therapy for TRT is based on this principle. As sound is added to the environment, the background activity in the auditory nervous system increases, which reduces the contrast between the tinnitus-related neuronal activity and the background activity. This reduced contrast has two results.*

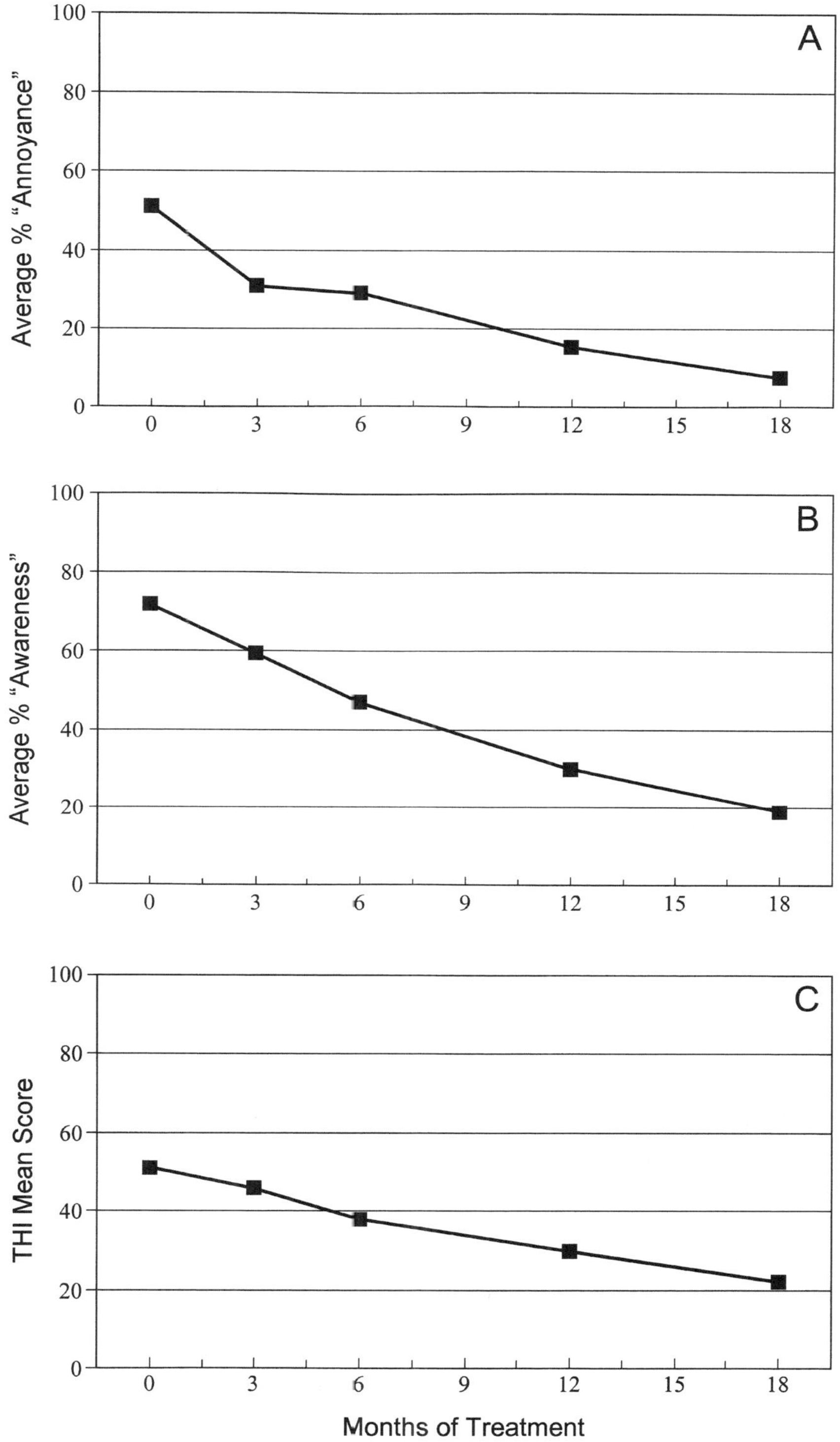

FIGURE 13–10. Data from a controlled clinical study showing the efficacy of TRT over a period of 18 months of treatment. **A.** Mean scores from the TRT Interview question *"What percent of your total awake time, over the last month, have you been* ***annoyed by*** *your tinnitus?"* **B.** Mean scores from the TRT Interview question *"What percent of your total awake time, over the last month, have you been* ***aware of*** *your tinnitus?"* **C.** Mean index scores from the Tinnitus Handicap Inventory (THI) (Newman, Jacobson, & Spitzer, 1996; Newman, Sandridge, & Jacobson, 1998). (Graph C adapted from *Clinical management of tinnitus using a "progressive intervention" approach* (p. 101) by Henry, J. A., Schechter, M. A., Loovis, C., Zaugg, T., Kaelin, C., & Montero, M. (2005). *Journal of Rehabilitation Research and Development, 42(Suppl. 2)*(4), 95–116. Adapted with permission from the author.)

First, the strength of the tinnitus signal connecting to the cortical and limbic areas of the brain is reduced. Second, detection of the tinnitus signal by subconscious neural networks becomes more difficult. Reducing detection of the tinnitus signal in this way facilitates the process of habituation, both of the reactions to tinnitus and of the perception of tinnitus.

Suppression of Tinnitus Is Counterproductive to Habituation

Sound can be used to suppress, or "mask," tinnitus, which is often done to achieve temporary relief from tinnitus. Suppression can be partial (changing the sound of the tinnitus) or complete (eliminating the perception of the tinnitus). Partial or complete suppression of tinnitus is counterproductive to achieving tinnitus habituation—which is the goal of TRT. Extinction of conditioned reflexes requires that the stimulus be present to learn that the stimulus is not reinforced. By definition, therefore, the extinction procedure for retraining the brain to habituate to the tinnitus requires that the tinnitus signal be unchanged.

Drugs and Tinnitus

It is the position of TRT that no prescription drug should be taken specifically for tinnitus, unless there is an emergency situation. [**Clinician:** TRT should not preclude the pharmacological management of patients with coexisting mental health issues. Also, effective implementation of TRT can result in a significant reduction in anxiety and depression inventory scores without the use of mood-altering medications.] *No drug has been shown to be consistently effective for tinnitus, and drugs often produce negative side effects* (Dobie, 1999). *Many patients do, however, take drugs for their tinnitus. These drugs usually target the central nervous system for management of anxiety; thus, they act to reduce activity in the limbic and autonomic nervous systems.*

Drugs Can Impair Learning

[**Clinician:** If a patient has been taking a drug for some time, it is not advised to stop taking the drug suddenly when treated with TRT.] *The use of drugs during treatment with TRT can slow the process of habituation if they impair central nervous system plasticity. This is especially an issue for benzodiazepines* (Kilic et al., 1999). [**Clinician:** There are other medications that do not impair plasticity/memory, e.g., drugs that act on glutamate receptors, calcium channels, and sodium channels. These kinds of drugs are worthy of future investigation and may prove to be synergistic with TRT.] *Just like drinking alcohol can impair the ability to learn, the use of benzodiazepines can interfere with the ability to learn, modify conditioned reflexes, think clearly, function normally, and participate in the mental and learning activities that are necessary with TRT.*

Habituation Takes Time

(Figure 13–10) *TRT is designed to promote habituation of reactions to tinnitus and habituation of perception of tinnitus. Both of these habituation processes normally require months, as the retraining occurs slowly and gradually. TRT involves a process of extinction of conditioned reflexes, which ideally would remove the negative reinforcement. As we discussed, in the case of tinnitus, the negative reinforcement cannot be removed completely during this process. Whereas some patients may experience improvement within 1 to 2 months, other patients require much longer. Most patients experience some habituation during the first 6 months of treatment. Regardless of the rate of progress, supervised treatment should take place for a minimum of 12 months to prevent relapse. Beyond 12 months, treatment continues until no further help is needed. During treatment there may be periods of rapid progress and periods of no perceptible progress. The TRT instructions should be followed closely regardless of what occurs during any given day.*

Summary

There are seven main summary points: (1) Perception of tinnitus is the result of normal compensation of the auditory system to some dysfunction or damage (typically occurring in the cochlea); (2) tinnitus becomes a problem only if it causes emotional reactions—simply perceiving tinnitus is not a problem; (3) the reactions caused by tinnitus are due mainly to conditioned reflexes; (4) treatment with TRT involves retraining conditioned reflexes, which is intended to result in habituation of the reactions caused by tinnitus, and habituation of the perception of tinnitus; (5) for habituation to occur, the brain must "reclassify" tinnitus as a neutral signal; (6) the proper use of sound will assist in the habituation process by decreasing the strength of the tinnitus signal; (7) the primary goal of TRT is habituation of the reactions caused by tinnitus—when the first goal is achieved, the secondary goal follows automatically: habituation of the perception of tinnitus.

SECTION 7: FITTING EAR-LEVEL DEVICES

[**Clinician:** If the patient is receiving sound generators or combination instruments, the devices are fitted and adjusted at this point during the counseling session. The fitting and adjustment procedures should be done in a reasonably quiet environment (the only time that quiet is recommended for TRT patients), but not in a sound-attenuated testing booth (which is an unrealistic acoustic environment). The clinician should first address any issues that would normally be covered as part of a hearing aid fitting (cleaning, care and maintenance, batteries, potentiometers, troubleshooting, etc.).

If the tinnitus is more bothersome in one side of the head or ear than the other, the sound generator (or combination instrument) should be placed in that ear first. If a combination instrument is being fitted, the output of the amplification portion should be adjusted prior to adjusting the level of the sound generator. The sound generator is normally adjusted to a level just below the "mixing point." The second device is then inserted. If the second device is a combination instrument, the amplification is first adjusted. The output of the second sound generator is then set to balance with the output of the first sound generator.]

What Is the "Mixing Point"?

[**Clinician:** It can be very difficult for patients to grasp the concept of the mixing point. The concept often needs to be explained and reexplained. This information should be covered thoroughly at the fitting appointment and at every return appointment.

Figure 13–11 shows that sound can cause three effects with respect to suppression of tinnitus: no suppression, partial suppression, and complete suppression. Patients can typically perceive all three suppression effects as the sound from their sound generators is gradually increased. Some patients, however, cannot distinguish all three effects. It is only critical for TRT patients to distinguish the mixing point, which is the threshold level between "no suppression" and "partial suppression."

At the lowest levels of the broadband noise, both the tinnitus and the noise can be heard clearly and distinctly. In this range (no suppression), the spectral characteristics of the tinnitus (i.e., quality or timbre of the tinnitus) are unchanged. Whether or not there is a difference (usually a reduction) in the perceived loudness of the tinnitus is irrelevant.

As the level of the noise is increased, the quality of the tinnitus sound starts to change at some point. Specifically, there are spectral changes in the tinnitus that are perceived by the patient. The level at which spectral changes in the tinnitus just start to occur defines the mixing point. The mixing point is the threshold level of the noise that is perceived by the patient to "mix," "blend," or "interfere" with the tinnitus (J. A. Henry, Zaugg, et al., 2005). At and above the mixing point (in the partial suppression range), the tinnitus can

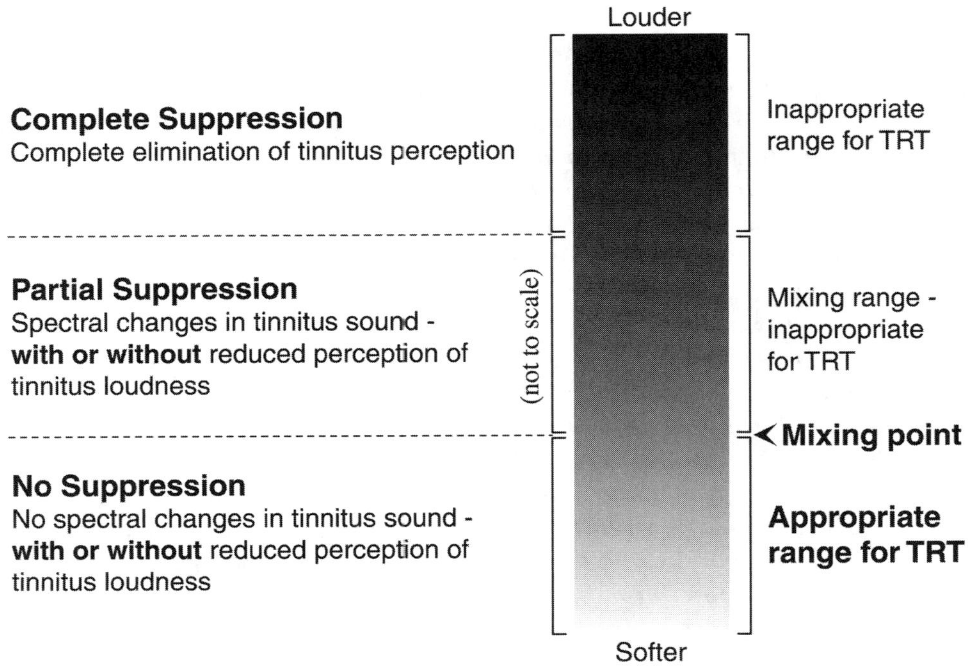

FIGURE 13–11. Effects of sound on tinnitus. This figure shows that as broadband noise is made louder, there are typically three ranges with respect to how the sound relates to the tinnitus. The lowest range is "no suppression." In this range, the sound does not affect the spectral characteristics of the tinnitus, i.e., the sound quality of the tinnitus does not change (the perceived tinnitus loudness may or may not change). The level of sound at which the tinnitus spectral characteristics start to change (with or without changes in perceived tinnitus loudness) is the "mixing point." Above the mixing point is the "partial suppression" range. As the sound is made still louder, it eventually causes "complete suppression" of the tinnitus. In this highest range, the tinnitus is inaudible. The only appropriate range for the use of sound with TRT is below the mixing point (in the no suppression range).

still be heard, but it is perceived to have different spectral characteristics. This change in tinnitus quality is not related to the perceived loudness of the tinnitus—there may or may not be a reduction in the perceived loudness.

As the noise is made louder in the partial suppression range, the tinnitus perception continues to change until the tinnitus can no longer be heard. This is the level at which "complete suppression" occurs.]

Adjusting Output of Sound Generators

[**Clinician:** With the concepts of sound therapy and the mixing point fully understood by the patient, the proper adjustment of sound generators is now explained in detail. (Note that the word *noise* should not be used when counseling patients because of its potential negative connotations. Instead, the word *sound* is always used in its place.) The patient should be aware that the output of the sound generators is adjusted every time the devices are placed in the ears—and at no other time. The level of the sound is adjusted initially to the mixing point, and then reduced slightly to be perceived below the mixing point (Figure 13–12).

It is very important to instruct patients that the sound from the devices should never create annoyance or discomfort, even if it is impossible to reach the mixing point. Inability to reach the mixing point, however, is secondary as there is a range of effective use of sound—referred to as

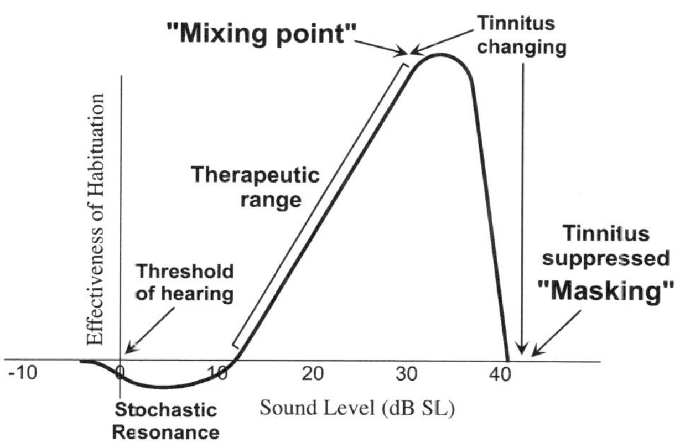

FIGURE 13–12. Theoretical function showing that the effectiveness of broadband noise for inducing habituation increases up to the "mixing point," i.e., up to the point at which the patient's tinnitus sound (timbre) changes and the noise and the tinnitus start to blend together audibly. As the level of the noise is increased, the tinnitus is suppressed (masked), which sharply reduces the potential for habituation. (Adapted from *Tinnitus Retraining Therapy: Implementing the Neurophysiological Model* (p. 115) by P. J. Jastreboff and J. W. P. Hazell, 2004, New York: Cambridge University Press. Copyright 2004 by Cambridge University Press. Adapted with permission from the author.)

the "therapeutic range" (Figure 13-12). The therapeutic range is above *stochastic resonance* and below the mixing point. Stochastic resonance refers to the effect that a signal, set close to the threshold of hearing, has on central auditory gain, which can theoretically enhance the tinnitus percept (P. J. Jastreboff, 1999b). For this reason, patients should be advised to not set the sound level very close to the threshold of audibility. At and above the mixing point, the tinnitus percept (timbre) changes, and this must not occur because patients cannot habituate to their "usual" tinnitus if the tinnitus percept is changed during sound therapy (Figure 13-11).

After the first sound generator is in place and adjusted to the proper level, the second sound generator is inserted and adjusted to match the perceived loudness of the sound generator in the first ear—disregarding the level of what might be a less bothersome tinnitus. (The less bothersome tinnitus may even be partially or completely suppressed in the process, which is acceptable.) The sound level in the second ear will be the same even if tinnitus is absent in this ear. If the sound level is too high (causing annoyance or suppressing the tinnitus), then it should be decreased in both devices to still be perceived as equally loud.]

Sound Generators: Points to Remember

[**Clinician:** These points are provided in Appendix C to use as a take-home reminder sheet for patients.] *Let's now review the **critical points** of using your ear-level devices: (1) Precise adjustment (within the therapeutic range) is optimal, providing that it is below the sound level that would cause annoyance or discomfort when the sound is used for many hours; (2) "Set and forget" (do not readjust the sound generators as long as they are worn continuously—readjustment attracts your attention to the devices, and may increase self-monitoring of the tinnitus, which is counterproductive to habituation); (3) Wear the devices every day and as often as possible (even while sleeping if desired); (4) Enrich your sound environment 24/7, whether wearing the devices or not; and (5) Return malfunctioning devices immediately for repair. The sound generators are normally used for 1 to 2 years, or until at least 2 or 3 months after you feel that they are no longer needed.*

TRT: Keys to Achieving Success

[**Note to clinician:** These points are provided in Appendix C.]

- Understand tinnitus and its benign nature
  - "Reclassify" tinnitus to the category of a neutral stimulus
- Avoid silence
- "Enrich" your sound environment 24/7
- Adjust and use sound generators according to the protocol
- Attend all follow-up appointments
- **With proper treatment**, habituation usually takes 1 to 2 years

14

Ongoing Treatment

Ongoing treatment is essential to perform TRT properly. All patients should be followed as necessary to ensure that they are fully compliant with every element of the treatment protocol and that they maintain an awareness of the principles of TRT counseling, which requires performing the counseling on a repeated basis over the course of treatment. The methodology for ongoing treatment, as described in this chapter, is mainly for Category 1 and 2 patients. Category 0 patients require a minimal protocol of counseling and follow-up (see Chapter 9). Category 3 and 4 patients require specific modifications to the ongoing treatment protocol, which are described in Chapter 15.

The present chapter explains the rationale for ongoing treatment and describes the appointment schedule, components of the appointments, and an abbreviated counseling protocol that can be used in lieu of the full TRT counseling protocol whenever it is not possible or necessary to perform all of the counseling. (It is emphasized that whenever the counseling is "abbreviated" or "minimal," the content of the counseling is not changed—it is only adjusted to a given category or to meet a patient's specific needs.) In addition, the TRT Follow-up Interview is explained, focusing on issues that are relevant to determining outcomes of treatment. Finally, suggestions are provided to address patients who do not make progress, and to determine the end point of treatment.

TRT directive counseling amounts to intense, repeated educational sessions for patients. Many new and technical concepts are introduced to patients. Patients have different retention abilities, but in general all patients need the counseling repeated so that the concepts can become firmly established in their minds. It is a general principle that learning is maximized through repetition. Studies have shown that patients retain only about 50% of the information received through educational counseling (Margolis, 2004; Shapiro, Boggs, Melamed, & Graham-Pole, 1992). Much of the information may be remembered incorrectly (Margolis, 2004), and as much as 80% of the information can be forgotten immediately (Kessels, 2003). Providing patients with take-home materials is thus also recommended.

Results of a controlled clinical trial support the need for ongoing treatment (J. A. Henry, Schechter, et al., 2005; J. A. Henry et al., 2006a, 2006b). In that study, repeated outcome measures were obtained at 3, 6, 12, and 18 months. The average responses of the TRT patients to these measures reveal a consistent progression of improvement at subsequent visits (Figure 13-10). Treatment progress actually may be minimal during the first 6 months of treatment with the greatest effects occurring after 6 months. These data strongly suggest that for TRT counseling to be optimally effective, it must be repeated at intervals over a period of at least a year (except for Category 0 patients who require only minimal counseling).

A general rule of thumb is that TRT patients should attend treatment appointments at 4 weeks, 3 months, 6 months, and then every 6 months until treatment is no longer needed (P. J. Jastreboff et al., 1996; P. J. Jastreboff & Hazell, 1993, 1998). During the first 3 months, contacts via telephone should be performed if there are no office visits during this period. Patients need to be fully aware of this schedule at the time they commit to the treatment program. Exceptions to this recommended schedule are necessary, of course, for patients who might need a greater amount of attention, or for those who are unable to make so many repeat visits. If travel poses a problem, counseling should at least be performed via telephone at the recommended intervals.

At every return appointment, ear-level devices should be checked for normal functioning, and patients should be queried as to their use and adjustment of the devices to ensure that they are complying with the device usage protocol.

TRT FOLLOW-UP INTERVIEW

The TRT Follow-up Interview and the Tinnitus Handicap Inventory (THI—see Chapter 8) are administered at all follow-up office visits and telephone consultations that adhere to the basic schedule of follow-up visits mentioned above. (It may be appropriate to administer them more often for patients who require additional treatment sessions.)

The Follow-up Interview contains a subset of questions from the Initial Interview. Some questions are essentially the same but are modified for the Follow-up Interview to monitor treatment progress and to determine outcomes of treatment. Both of these Interviews have been published in fully scripted versions along with descriptions of each question's intent (J. A. Henry et al., 2003). They are also available online (http://www.vard.org/jour/03/40/2/pdf/Henry.pdf). Updated versions of the Initial and Follow-up Interviews are provided in Appendices A and B, respectively.

Instructions to Patients

In the scripted initial instructions to the Follow-up Interview, patients are told to consider their tinnitus and its effects over the previous month when answering the questions. Patients are thus not asked to respond in relation to any particular day or circumstance, but to think of how the tinnitus has affected them generally during the prior 30 days. Clinicians should have their patients' previous responses available, and compare the current to the previous responses. Patients should not be informed of specific prior responses, but should be told if the responses indicate an improvement in their condition.

Tinnitus

Question 1

Question 1 in the Follow-up Interview contains a series of questions asking patients if they experience some days that are more affected by their tinnitus than others. The basic question about the number of "bad days" is asked in the Initial Interview (Question 7), and additional questions were added to the Follow-up Interview to determine if the number of bad days has changed relative to baseline. With positive results of treatment, patients will report fewer bad days than before. When asking these questions, clinicians should be aware if their patients are receiving treatment concurrently with anxiolytics or other psychotropic medications, and to take into account the potential effects of such treatment.

Questions 2–5

Questions 2 through 5 in the Follow-up Interview are the same as Questions 8 through 11, respectively, in the Initial Interview (see Chapter 10 and Appendix A). When obtaining these responses with the Follow-up Interview, clinicians should note any changes in patients' responses relative to the Initial Interview. It is particularly important to compare the response to Question 5 from the Follow-up Interview relative to Question 11 from the Initial Interview ("What is the biggest reason your tinnitus is a problem?"). The "biggest reason" that tinnitus is a problem can change from visit to visit, and the focus of counseling should be modified accordingly to address what the patient feels is the current primary concern.

Question 6

Question 6 determines the impact of tinnitus on various activities, as does Question 12 from the Initial Interview. Clinicians should have patients' responses to the Initial Interview in hand during administration of the Follow-up Interview. It is most helpful to write the previous responses on the Follow-up Interview form to enable direct comparisons during the questioning. Patients can be told if they have shown improvement or not but it is advised to not inform them of their previous responses, which helps to ensure that the responses are independent and unbiased.

Questions 7 and 8

Questions 7 and 8 address directly the main goals of treatment, which are habituation of perception and habituation of reactions, respectively, to tinnitus. These questions ask patients to estimate the percentage of their awake hours, over the previous month, that they were consciously aware of their tinnitus (tinnitus perception) and annoyed by their tinnitus (reactions to tinnitus). These percentages will decrease over time if treatment is successful in achieving habituation. The percentages will start out high at the beginning of treatment (often greater than 50%), and should gradually approach 0% as treatment progresses. Each of Questions 7 and 8 includes the additional questions (relative to the Initial Interview), "Has this percentage changed since the beginning of treatment?" (If "yes," "How much do you think it has changed?"). Patients' responses to the additional questions often contradict the actual differences in percentages between their Initial and Follow-up Interviews. Usually, when this occurs, patients are unaware of how much of a reduction has occurred over the course of treatment. When such a discrepancy occurs, this should be pointed out to the patient to emphasize the degree of progress that has been made.

Questions 9–11

Questions 9, 10, and 11 ask patients to report, respectively, their tinnitus loudness, tinnitus annoyance, and life impact due to their tinnitus on a 0-to-10 analog scale. (These questions are the same as Questions 15, 16, and 17 from the Initial Interview—please see the description of these questions in Chapter 10.) Each of these issues is particularly important with respect to outcomes of treatment. Patients may not be aware that improvement has occurred; thus, clinicians are again advised to have the patient's previous responses available to report any progress that has been made. An awareness of tangible progress can encourage patients and serve as an incentive to maintain full compliance with the treatment protocol to achieve optimal results.

Question 12

As treatment progresses, patients usually think differently about their tinnitus and how the tinnitus is affecting their lives. It is important to allow the patient sufficient opportunity to express any feelings about the tinnitus that may not have been covered in the previous questions. Most importantly, the patient's treatment category should be assessed to determine if it is still an appropriate placement. The treatment category can change during treatment, and the treatment must be modified accordingly if that occurs. Question 12 thus facilitates a discussion of these kinds of relevant concerns.

Sound Tolerance

Questions 13–22

The questions about sound tolerance in the Follow-up Interview are asked only if decreased sound tolerance was reported to be a problem during the Initial Interview. If sound tolerance was not a problem prior to treatment, then it is almost certainly not a problem at later visits (although there may be exceptions). Questions 13 through 22 in the Follow-up Interview are almost identical to Questions 19 through 30 in the Initial Interview. The main difference is that Question 14 also asks if there are any changes since the beginning of treatment with respect to "bad days" caused by decreased sound tolerance. For some of the questions, the clinician is advised to have the patient's responses to the Initial Interview available to compare the patient's perception of progress with the actual differences in the responses between the different Interview forms. It is important for patients to know that progress has been made, even if there is no perception of progress.

Hearing

Question 23

It is important at every appointment to determine if patients feel that they have a hearing problem. Question 23 in the Follow-up Interview addresses this issue. The key concern is the patient's *perception* of a hearing problem, regardless of the results of any auditory testing (Lutman, Brown, & Coles, 1987). If there is the perception of hearing difficulties, the patient probably requires amplification. This perception can change between appointments. Some patients who are marginal hearing aid candidates do not report a hearing problem during the initial assessment, but after using sound generators may report that hearing has since become problematic in some circumstances (J. A. Henry et al., 2006b). These patients may need their sound generators returned for combination instruments (or hearing aids); thus, it is important to make this determination very early in treatment. Any hearing difficulties during treatment will serve to frustrate the patient and ultimately can interfere with treatment outcomes.

Ranking Problems

Questions 24–26

Questions 24–26 are the same as Questions 34–36 from the Initial Interview. These questions all use the identical analog-scale format to assess the impact of tinnitus, decreased sound tolerance, and hearing loss on the patient's life. If more than one of these conditions is a problem for a patient, it is critical at every appointment to know how the patient ranks each problem in relation to the other problem(s). These relative rankings will often shift during treatment. A patient with an initially reported hearing problem should receive amplification, and the problem should be significantly reduced or eliminated at later appointments. If hyperacusis is initially the predominant problem, then it is treated first. When the hyperacusis problem is resolved, attention then focuses on the tinnitus (most hyperacusis patients also have tinnitus). Questions 24–26 are helpful in determining the main focus of treatment.

Question 27

Question 27 was added to the Follow-up Interview to ask patients if there have been any changes ("same," "better," or "worse") in their conditions of tinnitus, decreased sound tolerance, and hearing loss since the beginning of treatment. This question is of course asked only if multiple conditions are being treated. It is important to evaluate patients' subjective perception of change in relation to any numerical differences in the rankings between visits. (As already stated above, patients should be informed if improvement has occurred that is not readily apparent at the present visit.) A final question is asked with respect to the combined effects of the different conditions ("If you combine those issues, would you say your problem in general is the same, better, or worse than before you started treatment?").

Supplemental Questions

Question 28

This question asks patients how they would feel if they had to "give back" their ear-level devices. The question can be quite effective in assessing patients' true feelings about their devices. Patients may even become adamant (or defensive) in stating that they would not want to give up their instruments. The question is asked in an open-ended manner; i.e., the response choices are not mentioned to patients. The question often generates a discussion about the efficacy of the devices, which can be helpful to both patient and clinician. The response choice that is closest to the patient's statements is selected as the patient's response to the question.

Question 29

This final question in the TRT Follow-up Interview simply asks patients if they are glad that they started treatment. The patient's response provides a further indicator of the overall efficacy of treatment.

AUDIOMETRIC AND TINNITUS TESTING

The many articles written about TRT have generally recommended that all audiometric and tinnitus measures be repeated at the follow-up visits that occur at 6-month intervals (i.e., 6, 12, 18 months, etc.). Guidelines for performing this testing are provided in Chapter 11 (also see J. A. Henry, M. M. Jastreboff, et al., 2002). Some clinics, however, may not be able to perform all of the recommended testing. For example, Veterans Affairs medical centers in the United States do not function on a fee-per-service basis, and it may be difficult for them to justify so much testing when there is a long waiting list of patients (J. A. Henry, Schechter, Regelein, & Dennis, 2004). Therefore, a minimum amount of testing needs to be specified.

At each follow-up appointment, starting with the 3-month visit, the audiologist should at least obtain pure-tone audiometric thresholds. Other testing, including the tinnitus psychoacoustic assessment, should be conducted if indicated by patient report of any significant changes in auditory symptoms. For patients who reveal a loudness sensitivity problem at the initial evaluation, loudness discomfort levels (LDLs) should be repeated at all appointments until normal levels are observed. Remediation of loudness hypersensitivity is a goal of treatment with these patients, and LDL testing is necessary to note if there has been improvement.

COUNSELING

It should always be kept in mind that the purpose of TRT counseling is for patients to "reclassify" their tinnitus to the status of a benign, meaningless stimulus. This reclassification is necessary to initiate the process of habituation, and is also a prerequisite for achieving effectiveness with sound therapy.

The counseling protocol should be repeated at every major follow-up appointment (i.e., 1, 3, 6, 12, 18 months, etc.). There is, however, the important variable of patient comprehension ability that would affect how counseling is performed on an individual basis. For some patients it will be obvious at the follow-up appointments that they have a reasonably good grasp of the basic TRT principles (especially the neurophysiological model of tinnitus). For these patients, the counseling can be presented in an appropriately abbreviated manner, although all of the key principles should at least be mentioned to ensure that the patient has a clear understanding of the concepts (see next section). Other patients will have difficulty recalling the information, or they may have misunderstood the concepts during prior counseling. These latter patients will of course require extra time, and it may even be necessary to repeat everything from the initial counseling session.

Abbreviated Counseling Session

All patients, at some point during treatment, require only a review of the key TRT concepts. There are also instances when there is only time for a brief counseling session, or when patients call on the telephone and require a review of the counseling information. Further, Category 0 patients (who do not receive long-term treatment) may only require some very basic counseling (P. J. Jastreboff & Hazell, 2004). There is thus the need to specify the key concepts that would need to be covered during these shortened counseling sessions. Using the headings from the complete counseling protocol described in Chapter 13, topics are listed below that could be covered during such a brief session, which should require about 30 minutes to conduct. It may be helpful to provide a handout for patients to take home that contains a review of these principles. These concepts are listed below in the order in which they should be conveyed to patients, which is somewhat different from their order in the complete counseling protocol.

- Discordant Damage/Dysfunction
- Discordant Damage/Dysfunction Theory
- Auditory Gain
- The Heller and Bergman Experiment

- Why Is the Heller and Bergman Experiment Important?
- Perception of Signal Strength
- Perception of Tinnitus Strength
- What is the "Mixing Point"?
- Adjusting Output of Sound Generators
- Sound Generators: Points to Remember
- Section 5: Plasticity of the Brain
- Retraining of Conditioned Reflexes
- Section 6: The Neurophysiological Model of Tinnitus
- Conscious Loop
- Subconscious Loop
- Classification of New Sound: "Important"
- Reclassification of Sound: "Unimportant"
- Main Goal of Treatment with TRT
- Secondary Goal of Treatment with TRT
- Habituation and Passive Extinction
- Passive Extinction of Conditioned Reflexes
- Sound Therapy
- Reducing Contrast = Reducing Strength
- Habituation Takes Time
- Summary

TIME REQUIREMENTS TO CONDUCT FOLLOW-UP APPOINTMENTS

Follow-up Appointments Prior to 6 Months

Ideally, TRT patients should return at 4 weeks and 3 months following the initial treatment session. Some patients will require more appointments, and others may not be able to attend each of these appointments. For the 3-month visit, the time needed to perform the required tasks would include 10 to 15 minutes to check devices and ensure proper usage, 20 to 40 minutes to conduct the TRT Follow-up Interview, and up to 1 hour (or more) to conduct the counseling. The total time required for these appointments thus may reach 2 hours. Any other appointments conducted during the first 6 months of treatment, including the 4-week appointment, would generally be 30-minute appointments to answer questions, check devices, and ensure compliance with the protocol. However, some patients will require additional counseling, requiring substantial additional time.

Follow-up Appointments at 6-Month Intervals

The follow-up appointments conducted at 6-month intervals include, minimally, the same components as for the 3-month appointment, in addition to pure tone audiometric testing. Thus, as for the 3-month appointment, the time required to perform the minimum tasks at the 6-month-interval appointments is up to 2 hours—possibly longer due to the addition of threshold testing. At the later appointments, counseling time should be progressively reduced as patients become increasingly familiar with the information. Tinnitus loudness and pitch matching would add 10 to 15 minutes, and LDL testing would add about 10 to 20 minutes—if LDL testing is indicated by a sound tolerance problem. Repeating the complete audiometric and tinnitus testing would of course add even more time.

PATIENTS WHO DO NOT MAKE PROGRESS

Most patients who report minimal or no progress during treatment are simply unaware of their gradual progress over time, as indicated by a comparison of their responses between the Initial and Follow-up Interviews (and the repeated Tinnitus Handicap Inventory index scores). Some patients, however, will in fact not make progress, which will be corroborated by their interview and questionnaire responses. If little or no progress has been made after about 1 year of treatment, the clinician must make a full assessment of factors that could be hindering progress.

Some possible reasons for treatment failure include the following (P. J. Jastreboff & Hazell, 2004): (a) Patient was assigned to the wrong treatment category resulting in inappropriate treatment; (b) symptoms were temporarily worsened shortly after treatment started, and the patient was not properly counseled concerning the real nature of these effects; (c) patient did not fully comprehend the counseling information and thus reclassification of tinnitus to a neutral stimulus did not occur; (d) follow-up appointments were not made or were inadequate; (e) the neurophysiological model was not taught properly; (f) patient is involved in litigation, or is somehow receiving secondary benefit from the tinnitus (e.g., workers' compensation benefits); (g) severe psychological problems are untreated; (h) medications taken for psychiatric illness are exacerbating the tinnitus or impairing the brain's plasticity, which is necessary for habituation (specifically, all benzodiazepines can create significant problems); (i) strong need to attract attention ("flag wavers" describes patients who use their tinnitus or decreased sound tolerance as a pretext to attract attention and to ask for help). Each of these possibilities needs to be considered for the patient who is not showing progress. Obviously, these factors need to be checked and addressed properly at the initial stage of treatment. Delayed intervention decreases the chance of successful treatment.

Importantly, there is evidence that better health outcomes are associated with adherence to treatment (R. I. Horwitz & S. M. Horwitz, 1993). Treatment compliance is also a responsibility of the clinician; i.e., the clinician must ensure that the patient returns for counseling sessions according to the recommended treatment schedule. Patients also need to be queried carefully to make sure that they are using their ear-level devices according to the protocol. Anecdotally, J. A. Henry observed some subjects from a controlled study who reported that they were not making progress through about 1 year of treatment with TRT, but they continued to comply with the protocol and significant improvement was seen during the last period of treatment (J. A. Henry et al., 2006b). Additionally, P. J. Jastreboff observed a number of patients whose improvement appeared to be related to withdrawal from benzodiazepines. (Negative effects of antidepressants on tinnitus have not been observed.) In other cases, improvement was related to addressing misophonia in a more directed fashion. Some patients thus need to be encouraged to continue the treatment protocol in spite of their lack of progress.

It is important to recognize that the majority of patients would like to achieve a complete cessation of their tinnitus percept. This issue should be discussed with the patient prior to the initiation of treatment; otherwise the patient may never be satisfied. Decreased subjective perception of tinnitus loudness is generally observed in patients who successfully achieve even partial habituation of tinnitus. The neurophysiological model actually predicts this phenomenon as a side effect of decreased feedback from the limbic and autonomic nervous systems on the auditory nervous system (P. J. Jastreboff & M. M. Jastreboff, 2003). (Note that psychoacoustic loudness matches of tinnitus remain the same after the treatment.) Should the perception of tinnitus loudness fail to reduce, treatment can still be considered a success if and when significant habituation of reaction and perception is achieved based on history, rating scales, and overall quality of life reports.

It is possible that certain unpredictable tinnitus fluctuations will cause a renewed sense of concern that will require medical, surgical, and/or audiological evaluation and a possible repeat course of TRT, in which case habituation of reaction and perception can usually be achieved at a faster pace. Furthermore, achieving habituation of reaction and perception empowers the patient to optimally withstand and overcome potential future cyclical or noncyclical tinnitus fluctuations, especially if the change occurs gradually.

DETERMINING END OF TREATMENT

Treatment is completed when both the clinician and the patient agree that treatment is no longer necessary. This decision is facilitated by how the patient responds to the outcome questions in the TRT Follow-up Interview. These responses should indicate that tinnitus is no longer a clinically significant condition. Patients should not, however, stop using their sound generators at the time they first realize that their condition no longer requires treatment. If this occurs, patients should continue using their sound generators for at least 2 to 3 months to ensure that the retraining that has taken place is permanent. Treatment would of course also be terminated if a patient were no longer compliant with the follow-up schedule of appointments, or with the device usage protocol. When treatment is completed, patients should be advised to use their sound generators as needed anytime in the future should their tinnitus ever increase or become exacerbated. In the case of combination instruments a similar procedure is implemented for the sound generator portion of the instruments. Practically all patients with hearing aids will continue to use their hearing aids, but they are instructed that there is no need to provide additional sound enrichment as required during treatment.

15

Treatment For Decreased Sound Tolerance

Based on clinical data and experience, it is estimated that 25–30% of tinnitus patients have decreased sound tolerance to the extent that specific treatment is indicated (P. J. Jastreboff & Hazell, 2004). Conducting the Tinnitus Initial Interview and obtaining loudness discomfort levels (LDLs) will determine if the tinnitus patient has a significant problem with decreased sound tolerance, i.e., with inability to tolerate certain sounds that are tolerated comfortably by most other people. A sound tolerance problem usually consists of a combination of hyperacusis and misophonia (see Chapter 9). It is important to determine the presence of hyperacusis and misophonia as they each have a different impact on the treatment approach, and the protocols for their treatment are distinctly different. For example, if hyperacusis is a significant problem, then it should be the main focus of treatment. If misophonia creates a significant problem, then it can be treated concurrently with tinnitus.

Category 3 patients are diagnosed with hyperacusis. Hyperacusis refers to hypersensitivity to sound that is caused by abnormally strong reactions that are created within the auditory pathways. Subsequent activation of the limbic and autonomic nervous systems occurs due to the disproportionally high level of neuronal activity in the auditory pathways, which would normally be evoked by much louder sounds (e.g., neuronal activity evoked by 80 dB HL in a hyperacusis patient might be similar to activity evoked by 120 dB HL in an individual with normal loudness tolerance). Sounds causing these strong reactions can be soft or loud. The reactions are specific to the spectrum and intensity of the sound. Thus, sounds with similar acoustic characteristics would reliably cause similar reactions.

Whereas hyperacusis causes predictable physical reactions that are dictated by the spectrum and intensity of the offending sound, misophonic reactions may have little or nothing to do with the sound's acoustic characteristics. Misophonia is an aversion to certain sounds that is due to conditioned emotional responses (see Chapter 6) (P. J. Jastreboff & Hazell, 2004). Activity within the auditory system is within the norm, but enhanced functional connections between the auditory system and the limbic system for specific categories of stimuli result in strong activation of the limbic and autonomic nervous systems. Misophonic reactions depend on negative memories that are evoked when hearing sounds that are associated with negative experiences.

Most patients who are diagnosed with hyperacusis also experience some degree of misophonia, which further enhances activation of the limbic and autonomic nervous systems (see Figure 4–2). It is possible for some patients to experience only misophonia without a hyperacusis component. It has been reported that almost 60% of a population of 149 tinnitus patients experienced a sound tolerance problem, of which about half experienced misophonia without significant hyperacusis (i.e., without hyperacusis that required specific treatment) (M. M. Jastreboff & P. J. Jastreboff, 2002). In reality, it can be very difficult to make a clear distinction between effects due to hyperacusis versus those due to misophonia.

Phonophobia is a specific form of misophonia when fear is a dominant component of the patient's sound tolerance problem. Phonophobia is usually caused by irrational concerns that certain sounds will (a) cause damage to the auditory system, (b) exacerbate the tinnitus, and/or (c) cause physical pain.

Misophonic patients usually report that protective measures are used routinely to avoid exposure to uncomfortable sounds. These patients anticipate discomfort and typically *overprotect* their ears through the use of earplugs and/or earmuffs. The condition can become progressively worse due to the enhanced sensitivity caused by the overprotection (Formby & Gold, 2002).

Patients with *significant* hyperacusis are placed in TRT Category 3 (see Chapter 9). Note that misophonia does not affect the patient's TRT category, and patients with misophonia can be placed in any category depending on determining factors. P. J. Jastreboff and Hazell (2004) commented, "Note that hyperacusis should not be confused with misophonia or phonophobia; the latter can exist in any category and are treated concurrently with other problems by a separate protocol." Treatment for hyperacusis utilizes primarily a desensitization procedure involving the use of ear-level sound generators set at a comfortable level. Use of sound generators to treat hyperacusis should be continuous (i.e., during all waking hours, with some kind of bedside sound generator used during sleep time).

Category 3 patients who have a significant hearing loss requiring amplification will most likely have a problem tolerating sound that is amplified too much. For these patients, combination instruments (i.e., hearing aid combined with sound generator in one shell) are optimal, with the initial strategy being the use of sound generators with a low level of amplification and high compression. Alternatively, ear-level sound generators may be used at the initial stage for the desensitization process. With successful desensitization, amplification should be added at some point.

COUNSELING FOR DECREASED SOUND TOLERANCE

Counseling patients for hyperacusis always starts by covering the structured TRT counseling from the beginning of Section 1 through the Auditory Gain module in Section 2 (see Chapter 13). Most hyperacusis patients also have misophonia, and counseling should address both of these issues for these patients. Misophonia involves the same neural connections as for tinnitus, i.e., certain sounds activate the limbic system in the same way it is activated by a problem-tinnitus neural signal. Thus, the counseling for these patients should include an explanation of the neurophysiological model (from the perspective of "annoying sound" being the trigger of the reactions rather than tinnitus). Counseling for hyperacusis and misophonia also should include all of Section 5 (Plasticity of the Brain) and relevant portions of Section 6 (The Neurophysiological Model of Tinnitus). Clinicians should review Sections 5 and 6 and determine how best to adapt the materials to counsel for hyperacusis, misophonia, and phonophobia.

In addition, the companion counseling book (*Tinnitus Retraining Therapy: Patient Counseling Guide*) includes a supplementary section that is specific to counseling for hyperacusis (Section 8: Hyperacusis). As for the tinnitus counseling protocol provided in Chapter 13, a counseling protocol for hyperacusis is provided below that corresponds with Section 8 in the companion book. The scripted sections provide specific language that is suggested as a model for counseling patients. The script is based directly on the counseling protocol described by P. J. Jastreboff and Hazell (2004, Section 3.4.2, pp. 106–108), and emphasizes possible mechanisms underlying the condition.

Section 8: Hyperacusis

[**Clinician:** Prior to treating any condition of decreased sound tolerance, the terms hyperacusis, misophonia, and phonophobia need to be explained clearly to the patient. Thus, counseling for decreased sound tolerance begins with a differentiation of the concepts.]

Automatic Gain Control

The auditory system has automatic gain control. This means that the auditory system automatically modifies its sensitivity to sound according to the loudness of the sound being experienced at the time. This modification takes place both in the cochlea (peripherally) and in the central auditory pathways (centrally). When listening to very soft sounds, those sounds can be amplified as much as 60 dB by the outer hair cells. [**Clinician:** refer to Chapter 13, Hair Cell Loss: Outer versus Inner] *The central auditory pathways can amplify the signal even further. As the level of sound increases, this amplification decreases accordingly.*

Hyperacusis

(Figure 4–2) *Sometimes this gain mechanism provides too much amplification. When this occurs, sounds can seem abnormally loud. At some level the sounds become uncomfortably loud, or even painful. This would describe the condition of hyperacusis. A condition of "pure hyperacusis" would involve primarily the auditory pathways when overamplification occurs causing activation of the limbic and autonomic nervous systems. There is too much amplification taking place in the auditory system, which results in sounds being uncomfortably loud when they are comfortable for other people.*

Treating Hyperacusis

Assessment for hyperacusis involves testing for "loudness discomfort levels" and a detailed interview. During the testing, tones are made increasingly louder until they reach levels that are uncomfortably loud. A person with normal loudness tolerance will have an average loudness discomfort level around 100 dB HL or higher. With hyperacusis, loudness discomfort levels are reduced. The key to treating hyperacusis is to ***desensitize*** *the auditory system to sound. This involves systematic exposure to sounds that cause absolutely no annoyance. Over time, this results in the ability to listen comfortably to sounds that are gradually louder. Testing for loudness discomfort levels shows that these levels increase when the desensitization procedures are successful. Improvement in loudness tolerance can be observed in as little as a few weeks.*

Misophonia

(Figure 4–2) *Most patients with hyperacusis also have misophonia. Misophonia literally means "dislike of sound." Hyperacusis is the result of overamplification in the auditory system. In contrast, misophonia results from* ***emotional and autonomic reactions*** *to sounds. Thus, with misophonia the limbic and autonomic nervous systems are activated whenever a sound causes discomfort. These reactions are a result of conditioned reflexes. In other words, the brain learns to interpret certain sounds as uncomfortable or annoying. These sounds are annoying because they are associated with negative memories. When those memories are evoked by the sounds, there are emotional and autonomic (or stress) reactions to these sounds. Misophonia involves the same connections in the brain as for a tinnitus problem. These connections are between the auditory, limbic, and autonomic nervous systems, as shown in the neurophysiological model.*

Treating Misophonia

(Figure 4–2) *To treat misophonia, the connections between the auditory, limbic, and autonomic nervous systems that cause the emotional reactions must be* ***retrained****. This retraining occurs by active extinction of conditioned reflexes that are responsible for the reactions to sounds. This is accomplished by consistently creating a positive association with sound by, for example, listening to pleasant sound while paying attention to it. The key is to* ***listen*** *to these sounds, which is different from having sounds in the background that are essentially ignored. This* ***active listening*** *process results in positive feelings about listening to these sounds, which is what extinguishes the conditioned reflexes.* [**Clinician:** Note that this recommendation is the opposite of what is recommended for hyperacusis when sounds need to be neutral and patients are instructed to ignore them and not to listen to them.] *Usually, hyperacusis and misophonia occur together. Thus, the treatment should include both desensitization of the auditory system to address the hyperacusis, and active listening to pleasant sounds to address the misophonia.*

Phonophobia

Phonophobia is a specific type of misophonia that involves ***fear of sound****. Misophonia results in emotional reactions to sound, and the condition is not phonophobia if there is no fear involved in the reaction. Sometimes, people with tinnitus or hyperacusis become fearful that certain sounds can cause damage to the auditory system or cause the hyperacusis or tinnitus to become worse. This would be the typical reason that a fear response would develop. As a result of the fear, these people overprotect their ears to avoid worsening their condition. They either use hearing protection (earplugs and/or earmuffs) or avoid the sounds altogether. These sounds that are feared, however, are generally harmless. Overprotecting the ears can make the auditory system even more sensitive, which is what can actually worsen the condition. Treatment for phonophobia involves specific counseling regarding the benign nature of any sound that causes a phonophobic reaction, and that the auditory system needs sound for normal functioning. The identical sound-therapy protocol is used for phonophobia as for misophonia.*

ONGOING TREATMENT

Effects of treatment for hyperacusis can be observed in a period of weeks, and the problem can often be resolved in a period of months. In some cases it is possible to achieve a total cure for hyperacusis and/or misophonia. The time period for improvement depends on many factors, but the important point is that treatment for hyperacusis should occur on a different schedule than for tinnitus. The schedule should depend mainly on the severity of the problem. Patients with a particularly severe condition should be seen every week. Patients with moderate severity might be seen every 2–3 weeks. These intervals should be maintained only as long as necessary. Once the hyperacusis is under control, the emphasis of treatment should shift to addressing the tinnitus problem (which is the case for most hyperacusis patients). In the case of misophonia, the treatment schedule follows the typical protocol as for Category 1 and 2 tinnitus patients, as described in Chapter 14.

Monitoring the progress of treatment for hyperacusis involves testing LDLs (Chapter 11) and administering the TRT Follow-up Interview (Chapter 14 and Appendix B). Testing for LDLs and administering the Follow-up Interview should be done at every appointment for these patients. Obtaining LDLs can help to document any reported change in sound tolerance, and will assist in determining the level of sound that can be used for treatment (P. J. Jastreboff & Hazell, 2004). Testing of LDLs can be an uncomfortable experience for some patients, and this testing should be done with extreme caution, postponed, and/or avoided in some circumstances.

TREATING CATEGORY 4 PATIENTS

As described in Chapter 9, Category 4 patients experience exacerbation of tinnitus and/or hyperacusis that is still experienced after a night's sleep following exposure to certain environmental sounds. The effect can last days or even weeks. It is critical that these patients receive appropriate treatment "because inappropriate treatment can have devastating results" (P. J. Jastreboff & Hazell, 2004, p. 131).

Most Category 4 patients have hyperacusis as their dominant problem; thus, the hyperacusis counseling protocol described above should be completed (P. J. Jastreboff & Hazell, 2004). The treatment strategy focuses on the presentation of sound at the highest tolerable levels above threshold (which are usually very low) without producing the *winding-up* or *kindling* effects. (Recall from Chapter 9 that winding-up refers to the phenomenon whereby tinnitus and/or hyperacusis are exacerbated for a prolonged period of time due to exposure to some continuous sound, while kindling describes the situation when exposure to sound does not initially create discomfort but after several repetitions starts to evoke discomfort.) It is important to differentiate real Category 4 patients from patients with strong misophonia as they can exhibit similar behavior. Patients with Lyme disease, head injury, and neurological problems are more prone to be assigned to Category 4. The primary aim of treatment is to desensitize the auditory pathways in a manner similar to the treatment of hyperacusis patients. Concerns about inducing stochastic resonance are secondary—it may be necessary to use sound at near-threshold levels to start the desensitization process. However, patients should be carefully counseled about the stochastic resonance effect (using Figure 13-12) so that they are fully aware of the potential effects of sound at different levels relative to threshold. The most conservative method of sound presentation for these patients, with the least risk of tinnitus or hyperacusis exacerbation, is to start at low suprathreshold levels, and to very gradually increase the levels over time.

More specifically, Category 4 patients are fitted with binaural ear-level sound generators and instructed to adjust the sound output close to threshold for the first few weeks (P. J. Jastreboff & Hazell, 2004). If patients seem to experience global hypersensitivity, they may need a week or so just to get used to the devices being worn in their ears, in which case the devices may be worn without being switched on. Treatment then progresses to consecutive periods ("blocks") of 6–8 weeks that each involve a slight increase in the level of sound presented from the sound generators. If the tinnitus or hyperacusis becomes exacerbated during any of these blocks, then the level is reduced to the level from the previous block. It is critical that patients use the sound generators continuously throughout each day.

Category 4 patients are the most difficult patients to achieve treatment success with TRT. When outcomes are positive, recovery generally takes longer than for the other categories. Further information about treating this challenging and unpredictable group of patients can be found in P. J. Jastreboff & Hazell (2004, especially pp. 131–133).

16

Summary and Conclusion

Tinnitus is one stimulus in a "sea of stimuli." With chronic tinnitus, the stimulus is present constantly—other sensory stimuli are temporary and circumstantial. Most people afflicted with tinnitus ignore it most of the time—they have habituated to their tinnitus just like they habituate naturally to insignificant sounds. Some people, however, attend consciously to their tinnitus much of the time. Directed attention given to tinnitus increases the likelihood of reacting negatively to it. Once these negative reactions start occurring, they are difficult to stop and can be debilitating. The problem is not the tinnitus itself, but the *reactions* to it. If a tinnitus sufferer can stop reacting to the tinnitus (habituation of reaction), the tinnitus perception time will diminish (habituation of perception) accordingly and the tinnitus will cease being a problem and the suffering will end.

Although neural mechanisms of tinnitus are not yet fully understood, many insights can be gained through a careful examination of what is known about the neurophysiology of the auditory nervous system. By applying what is known about neural auditory processing, many aspects of tinnitus as an auditory percept can be reasonably theorized. P. J. Jastreboff's neurophysiological model depicts tinnitus as neural activity in the auditory nervous system, with other parts of the CNS (cortical, limbic, and autonomic nervous systems) involved in those persons for whom tinnitus becomes annoying or intrusive—approximately 20% of all individuals who experience constant tinnitus. For this subgroup, a vicious circle of positive feedback is described by the model as a progressive enhancement of cortical, limbic, and autonomic activity that is triggered by the tinnitus-related neural signal. Because of what the tinnitus patient has "learned" in the development of this vicious circle, retraining must take place to deactivate the autonomic and limbic responses and to block the tinnitus signal from reaching cortical areas of awareness. Achieving these goals is largely dependent upon the clinician's effectiveness in providing the counseling and orchestrating the appropriate sound therapy (and auditory rehabilitation if needed). These are the essential concepts upon which TRT counseling is based and that establish the foundation for TRT therapists. As patients continue to learn and grasp the neurophysiological model of tinnitus and the intricate role that the brain plays in modulating the tinnitus signal, compliance with therapy increases. As a result, hope, control, and relief are obtained, and the realistic goal of long-term habituation is achieved.

It can be a daunting task for the tinnitus sufferer to find a competent tinnitus practitioner. There are numerous methodologies for treating tinnitus, most of which involve counseling and/or the use of sound for therapy (Tyler, 2005). At this time it is not possible to state unequivocally that there is one method of treatment that works best for all patients. In defense of TRT, our controlled clinical trial has shown that treatment with TRT, when done properly by a trained and experienced professional, can be very effective for the majority of patients treated (J. A. Henry, Schechter, et al., 2005; J. A. Henry et al., 2006a, 2006b). The reader who is interested in the clinical and research evidence for TRT is advised to review Chapter 4 in the original book about TRT (P. J. Jastreboff & Hazell, 2004).

The intent of the present book is to provide clinicians with a practical and detailed guide to evaluate and treat their tinnitus patients with TRT. The book supplements many previous articles about TRT, the original TRT book, and the TRT instructional courses. What sets this book apart is the detailed clinical procedures that are described, as well as the unique perspectives on the neurophysiological model and other aspects of the TRT paradigm.

Although it is essential to conduct TRT according to the specified protocol, it has been observed that some clinicians modify the procedures, usually by inappropriately abbreviating the counseling or by not providing the requisite follow-up care. Because of the specificity of the protocol, TRT should be practiced with minimal variation, ensuring that every patient receives the same standard of treatment.

This book, along with the companion book, represents an attempt to present a clear description of procedures to conduct assessment and treatment with TRT. With study and experience in applying these techniques, clinicians can become facile in conducting TRT and can be an effective resource for their patients. The effectiveness of TRT also depends on the clinician exhibiting a compassionate and unhurried attitude, and expressing confidence and hope in the outcome of treatment. The goal is to empower patients to gain control over their tinnitus and to ultimately experience relief that will help them reclaim a lifestyle unhindered by tinnitus.

References

Abel, J. R. (1999). *The eye care revolution: Prevent and reverse common vision problems*. New York: Kennington.

Allan, R. W. (1998). Operant-respondent interactions. In W. O'Donohue (Ed.), *Learning and behavior therapy* (pp. 146–168). Needham Heights, MA: Allyn & Bacon.

Amaral, D. G. (2000). The anatomical organization of the central nervous system. In E. R. Kandel, J. H. Schwartz, & T. M. Jessell (Eds.), *Principles of neural science* (pp. 318–336). New York: McGraw-Hill.

Anderson, J. A. (1995). *An introduction to neural networks*. Cambridge, MA: The MIT Press.

American Speech-Language-Hearing Association. (2004). Scope of practice in audiology. *ASHA Suppl. 24* (in press).

Axelsson, A., & Barrenas, M.-L. (1992). Tinnitus in noise-induced hearing loss. In A. L. Dancer, D. Henderson, R. J. Salvi, & R. P. Hamnernik (Eds.), *Noise-induced hearing loss* (pp. 269–276). St. Louis, MO: Mosby-Year Book.

Axelsson, A., & Ringdahl, A. (1989). Tinnitus: A study of its prevalence and characteristics. *British Journal of Audiology*, *23*, 53–62.

Basbaum, A. I., & Jessell, T. M. (2000). The perception of pain. In E. R. Kandel, J. H. Schwartz, & T. M. Jessell (Eds.), *Principles of neural science* (4th ed., pp. 472–491). New York: McGraw-Hill.

Bauer, C. A. (2004). Mechanisms of tinnitus generation. *Current Opinions in Otolaryngology Head and Neck Surgery*, *12*(5), 413–417.

Beattie, R. C., & Sheffler, M. V. (1981). Test-retest reliability and effects of psychophysical methods on the speech loudness discomfort level. *Audiology*, *20*, 143–156.

Beck, A. T., Ward, C. H., Mendelson, M., Mock, J., & Erbaugh, J. (1961). An inventory for measuring depression. *Archives of General Psychiatry*, *4*, 561–571.

Brodal, P. (2004). *The central nervous system: Structure and function*. New York: Oxford University Press.

Burns, E. M. (1984). A comparison of variability among measurements of subjective tinnitus and objective stimuli. *Audiology*, *23*, 426–440.

Byrne, D., & Dirks, D. (1996). Effects of acclimatization and deprivation on non-speech auditory abilities. *Ear and Hearing*, *17*(3 Suppl.), 29S–37S.

Cacace, A. T. (2003). Expanding the biological basis of tinnitus: Crossmodal origins and the role of neuroplasticity. *Hearing Research*, *175*(1–2), 112–132.

Cacace, A. T. (2004). The limbic system and tinnitus. In J. B. Snow (Ed.), *Tinnitus: Theory and management* (pp. 162–170). Hamilton, Ontario: BC Decker.

Carhart, R., & Jerger, J. F. (1959). Preferred method for clinical determination of pure-tone thresholds. *Journal of Speech and Hearing Disorders*, *24*, 330–345.

Carlson, N. R. (1991). *Physiology of behavior*. Needham Heights, MA: Allyn and Bacon.

Chapman, P. F., & Chattarji, S. (2000). Synaptic plasticity in the amygdala. In J. P. Aggleton, (Ed.), *The amygdala: A functional analysis.* (pp. 117–153). New York: Oxford University Press.

Chen, G. D., & Jastreboff, P. J. (1995). Salicylate-induced abnormal activity in the inferior colliculus of rats. *Hearing Research*, *82*(2), 158–178.

Chole, R. A., & Parker, W. S. (1992). Tinnitus and vertigo in patients with temporomandibular disorder. *Archives of Otolaryngology, Head and Neck Surgery*, *118*(8), 817–821.

Clark, J. C., & Martin, F. N. (1994). *Effective counseling in audiology*. Upper Saddle River, NJ: Prentice-Hall.

Coles, R. R. A. (1995). Classification of causes, mechanisms of patient disturbance, and associated counseling. In J. A. Vernon & A. R. Moller (Eds.), *Mechanisms of Tinnitus* (pp. 11–19). Needham Heights, MA: Allyn & Bacon.

Coles, R. R. A. (1996). Tinnitus: Epidemiology, aetiology and classification. In G. Reich & J. A. Vernon (Eds.), *Proceedings of the Fifth International Tinnitus Seminar 1995* (pp. 25–29). Portland, OR: American Tinnitus Association.

Davis, A., & Refaie, A. E. (2000). Epidemiology of tinnitus. In R. Tyler (Ed.), *Tinnitus handbook* (pp. 1–23). San Diego, CA: Singular Publishing Group.

Davis, M. (2000). The role of the amygdala in conditioned and unconditioned fear and anxiety. In J. P. Aggleton (Ed.), *The amygdala: A functional analysis* (pp. 213–287). New York: Oxford University Press.

Daw, N. D., Kakade, S., & Dayan, P. (2002). Opponent interactions between serotonin and dopamine. *Neural Networks, 15*(4–6), 603–616.

Department of Veterans Affairs. (2005). *Screening for PTSD in a primary care setting*. Retrieved January 27, 2007, from http://www.ncptsd.va.gov/ncmain/index.jsp

Dobie, R. A. (1999). A review of randomized clinical trials in tinnitus. *The Laryngoscope, 109*, 1202–1211.

Dobie, R. A. (2002). Randomized clinical trials for tinnitus: Not the last word? In R. Patuzzi (Ed.), *Proceedings of the Seventh International Tinnitus Seminar* (pp. 3–6). Crawley: The University of Western Australia.

Dobie, R. A. (2004a). Clinical trials and drug therapy for tinnitus. In J. B. Snow (Ed.), *Tinnitus: Theory and management* (pp. 266–277). Lewiston, NY: BC Decker.

Dobie, R. A. (2004b). Overview: Suffering from tinnitus. In J. B. Snow (Ed.), *Tinnitus: Theory and management* (pp. 1–7). Lewiston, NY: BC Decker.

Dobie, R. A., & Sullivan, M. D. (1998). Antidepressant drugs and tinnitus. In J. A. Vernon (Ed.), *Tinnitus treatment and relief* (pp. 43–51). Needham Heights, MA: Allyn & Bacon.

Domjan, M., & Burkhard, B. (1986). *The principles of learning and behavior*. Pacific Grove, CA: Brooks/Cole.

Doron, N. N., & LeDoux, J. E. (1999). Organization of projections to the lateral amygdala from auditory and visual areas of the thalamus in the rat. *Journal of Comparative Neurology, 412*(3), 383–409.

Eggermont, J. J., & Roberts, L. E. (2004). The neuroscience of tinnitus. *Trends in Neuroscience, 27*(11), 676–682.

Erlandsson, S. (2000). Psychological profiles of tinnitus patients. In R. S. Tyler (Ed.), *Tinnitus Handbook* (pp. 25–57). San Diego, CA: Singular Publishing Group.

Erlandsson, S. I., Hallberg, L. R. M., & Axelsson, A. (1992). Psychological and audiological correlates of perceived tinnitus severity. *Audiology, 31*, 168–179.

Falls, W. A. (1998). Extinction: A review of theory and the evidence suggesting that memories are not erased with nonreinforcement. In W. O'Donohue (Ed.), *Learning and behavior therapy* (pp. 205–299). Needham Heights, MA: Allyn & Bacon.

Feng, H.-J., & Faingold, C. L. (2002). Repeated generalized audiogenic seizures induce plastic changes on acoustic evoked neuronal firing in the amygdala. *Brain Research, 932*, 61–69.

Folmer, R. L., & Griest, S. E. (2000). Tinnitus and insomnia. *American Journal of Otolaryngology, 21*(5), 287–293.

Formby, C., & Gold, S. L. (2002). Modification of loudness discomfort level: Evidence for adaptive chronic auditory gain and its clinical relevance. *Seminars in Hearing, 23*, 21–35.

Formby, C., Sherlock, L. P., & Gold, S. L. (2002). Adaptive recalibration of chronic auditory gain: Interim findings. In R. Patuzzi (Ed.), *Proceedings of the Seventh International Tinnitus Seminar* (pp. 165–169). Crawley: The University of Western Australia.

Fowler, E. P. (1942). The "illusion of loudness" of tinnitus—Its etiology and treatment. *Laryngoscope, 52*, 275–285.

Fuster, J. M. (1989). *The prefrontal cortex*. New York: Raven.

Gagne, J.-P. (1998). Reflections on evaluative research in audiological rehabilitation. *Scandinavian Audiology, 27*(Suppl. 49), 69–79.

Gardner, E. P., & Martin, J. H. (2000). Coding of sensory information. In E. R. Kandel, J. H. Schwartz, & T. M. Jessell (Eds.), *Principles of neural science* (pp. 411–429). New York: McGraw-Hill.

Garnes, S. J., & Pinel, J. P. J. (2001). Conditioned effects of kindling. *Neuroscience and Behavioral Reviews, 25*, 745–751.

Gilman, S., & Newman, S. W. (2003). *Manter and Gatz's essentials of clinical neuroanatomy and neurophysiology* (10th ed.). Philadelphia: F. A. Davis.

Gitt, W. (1999). *The wonder of man*. Bielefeld, Germany: Christliche Literatur-Verbreitung.

Gold, S. L., Frederick, E. A., & Formby, C. (1999). Shifts in dynamic range for hyperacusis patients receiving tinnitus retraining therapy (TRT). In J. Hazell (Ed.), *Proceedings of the Sixth International Tinnitus Seminar 1999* (pp. 297–301). London: The Tinnitus and Hyperacusis Centre.

Gordon-Salant, S. (2005). Hearing loss and aging: New research findings and clinical implications. *Journal of Rehabilitation Research and Development, 42*(4 Suppl. 2), 9–24.

Graham, J. T., & Newby, H. A. (1962). Acoustical characteristics of tinnitus: An analysis. *Archives of Otolaryngology, 75*, 82–87.

Hallam, R., Rachman, S., & Hinchcliffe, R. (1984). Psychological aspects of tinnitus. In S. Rachman (Ed.), *Contributions to medical psychology* (Vol. 3, pp. 31-53). Oxford: Pergamon Press.

Hawkins, D. B., Walden, B., & Montgomery, A. (1987). Description and validation of an LDL procedure designed to select SSPL90. *Ear and Hearing, 8*, 162-169.

Hazell, J. W. P. (1995). Models of tinnitus: Generation, perception, clinical implications. In J. A. Vernon & A. R. Møller (Eds.), *Mechanisms of tinnitus* (pp. 57-72). Needham Heights, MA: Allyn & Bacon.

Hazell, J. W. P. (1996a). Support for a neurophysiological model of tinnitus. In G. E. Reich & J. A. Vernon (Eds.), *Proceedings of the Fifth International Tinnitus Seminar* (pp. 51-57). Portland, OR: American Tinnitus Association.

Hazell, J. W. P. (1996b). Tinnitus as a manifestation of a survival style reflex. In G. E. Reich & J. A. Vernon (Eds.), *Proceedings of the Fifth International Tinnitus Seminar* (pp. 579-588). Portland, OR: American Tinnitus Association.

Hazell, J. W. P. (1998). Management of tinnitus. In H. Ludman & T. Wright (Eds.), *Diseases of the ear* (pp. 202-215). London: Arnold.

Hazell, J. W. P. (1999). The TRT method in practice. In J. Hazell (Ed.), *Proceedings of the Sixth International Tinnitus Seminar 1999* (pp. 92-98). London: The Tinnitus and Hyperacusis Centre.

Hazell, J. W. P. (2002). Tinnitus retraining therapy based on the Jastreboff model. http://www.tinnitus.org.

Hazell, J. W. P., & Sheldrake, J. B. (1992). Hyperacusis and tinnitus. In J.-M. Aran & R. Dauman (Eds.), *Tinnitus 91: Proceedings of the Fourth International Tinnitus Seminar* (pp. 245-248). Amsterdam/New York: Kugler Publications.

Heller, M. F., & Bergman, M. (1953). Tinnitus aurium in normally hearing persons. *Annals of Otology, 62*, 73-83.

Henry, J. A. (2004). Audiologic assessment. In J. B. Snow (Ed.), *Tinnitus: Theory and management* (pp. 220-236). Lewiston, NY: BC Decker.

Henry, J. A., Dennis, K., & Schechter, M. A. (2005). General review of tinnitus: Prevalence, mechanisms, effects, and management. *Journal of Speech, Language, and Hearing Research, 48*(5), 1204-1234.

Henry, J. A., Fausti, S. A., Mitchell, C. R., Flick, C. L., Helt, W. J., & Ellingson, R. M. (2000). Computer-automated clinical technique for tinnitus quantification. *American Journal of Audiology, 9*, 36-49.

Henry, J. A., Flick, C. L., Gilbert, A. M., Ellingson, R. M., & Fausti, S. A. (2001). Comparison of two computer-automated procedures for tinnitus pitch matching. *Journal of Rehabilitation Research and Development, 38*, 557-566.

Henry, J. A., Flick, C. L., Gilbert, A. M., Ellingson, R. M., & Fausti, S. A. (2004). Comparison of manual and computer-automated procedures for tinnitus pitch-matching. *Journal of Rehabilitation Research and Development, 41*(2), 121-138.

Henry, J. A., Flick, C. L., Gilbert, A. M., Ellingson, R. M., Silaski, G. C., & Fausti, S. A. (1999). Fully-automated system for tinnitus loudness and pitch matching. In J. Hazell (Ed.), *Proceedings of the Sixth International Tinnitus Seminar* (pp. 520-521). Cambridge, UK: The Tinnitus and Hyperacusis Centre.

Henry, J. A., Jastreboff, M. M., Jastreboff, P. J., Schechter, M. A., & Fausti, S. A. (2002). Assessment of patients for treatment with Tinnitus Retraining Therapy. *Journal of the American Academy of Audiology, 13*, 523-544.

Henry, J. A., Jastreboff, M. M., Jastreboff, P. J., Schechter, M. A., & Fausti, S. A. (2003). Guide to conducting Tinnitus Retraining Therapy (TRT) Initial and Follow-up Interviews. *Journal of Rehabilitation Research and Development, 40*, 157-178.

Henry, J. A., & Meikle, M. B. (2000). Psychoacoustic measures of tinnitus. *Journal of the American Academy of Audiology, 11*, 138-155.

Henry, J. A., Schechter, M. A., Loovis, C., Zaugg, T., Kaelin, C., & Montero, M. (2005). Clinical management of tinnitus using a "progressive intervention" approach. *Journal of Rehabilitation Research and Development, 42*(Suppl. 2)(4), 95-116.

Henry, J. A., Schechter, M. A., Nagler, S. M., & Fausti, S. A. (2002). Comparison of Tinnitus Masking and Tinnitus Retraining Therapy. *Journal of the American Academy of Audiology, 13*, 559-581.

Henry, J. A., Schechter, M. A., Regelein, R. T., & Dennis, K. C. (2004). Veterans and tinnitus. In J. B. Snow (Ed.), *Tinnitus: Theory and management* (pp. 337-355). Lewiston, NY: BC Decker.

Henry, J. A., Schechter, M. A., Zaugg, T. L., Griest, S. E., Jastreboff, P. J., Vernon, J. A., et al. (2006a). Clinical trial to Compare Tinnitus Masking and Tinnitus Retraining Therapy. *Acta Oto-Laryngologica, 126, Suppl. 556,* 64-69.

Henry, J. A., Schechter, M. A., Zaugg, T. L., Griest, S. E., Jastreboff, P. J., Vernon, J. A., et al. (2006b). Outcomes of clinical trial: Tinnitus Masking vs. Tinnitus Retraining Therapy. *Journal of the American Academy of Audiology, 17*, 104-132.

Henry, J. A., Zaugg, T., & Schechter, M. A. (2005). Clinical guide for audiologic tinnitus management I: Assessment. *American Journal of Audiology, 14*, 21-48.

Henry, J. L., & Wilson, P. H. (1998). Psychological treatments for tinnitus. In J. A. Vernon (Ed.), *Tinnitus treatment and relief* (pp. 99-115). Needham Heights, MA: Allyn & Bacon.

Henry, J. L., & Wilson, P. H. (2001). *The psychological management of chronic tinnitus*. Needham Heights, MA: Allyn & Bacon.

Hodgson, W. R. (1994a). Audiologic counseling. In J. Katz (Ed.), *Handbook of clinical audiology* (4th ed., pp. 616–623). Baltimore: Williams & Wilkins.

Hodgson, W. R. (1994b). Evaluating infants and young children. In J. Katz (Ed.), *Handbook of clinical audiology* (4th ed., pp. 465–475). Baltimore: Williams & Wilkins.

Horwitz, R. I., & Horwitz, S. M. (1993). Adherence to treatment and health outcomes. *Archives of Internal Medicine*, *153*(16), 1863–1868.

Hu, B. (2003). Functional organization of lemniscal and nonlemniscal auditory thalamus. *Experimental Brain Research*, *153*(4), 543–549.

Iversen, S., Iversen, L., & Saper, C. B. (2000). The autonomic nervous system and the hypothalamus. In E. R. Kandel, J. H. Schwartz, & T. M. Jessell (Eds.), *Principles of neural science* (pp. 960–981). New York: McGraw-Hill.

Iversen, S., Kupfermann, I., & Kandel, E. R. (2000). Emotional states and feelings. In E. R. Kandel, J. H. Schwartz, & T. M. Jessell (Eds.), *Principles of neural science* (pp. 982–997). New York: McGraw-Hill.

Jakes, S. C., Hallam, R. S., Chambers, C., & Hinchcliffe, R. (1985). A factor analytical study of tinnitus complaint behaviour. *Audiology*, *24*, 195–206.

Jakes, S. C., Hallam, R. S., Rachman, S., & Hinchcliffe, R. (1986). The effects of reassurance, relaxation training and distraction on chronic tinnitus sufferers. *Behaviour Research and Therapy*, *24*, 497–507.

Jastreboff, M. M. (1999). Controversies between cognitive therapies and TRT counseling. In J. Hazell (Ed.), *Proceedings of the Sixth International Tinnitus Seminar 1999* (pp. 288–291). London: The Tinnitus and Hyperacusis Centre.

Jastreboff, M. M., & Jastreboff, P. J. (1999). Questionnaires for assessment of the patients and their outcomes. In J. W. P. Hazell (Ed.), *Proceedings of the Sixth International Tinnitus Seminar 1999* (pp. 487–491). London: The Tinnitus and Hyperacusis Centre.

Jastreboff, M. M., & Jastreboff, P. J. (2002). Decreased sound tolerance and Tinnitus Retraining Therapy (TRT). *Australian and New Zealand Journal of Audiology*, *24*, 74–81.

Jastreboff, P. J. (1981). Cerebellar interaction with the acoustic reflex. *Acta Neurobiology Experiments*, *41*(3), 279–298.

Jastreboff, P. J. (1990). Phantom auditory perception (tinnitus): Mechanisms of generation and perception. *Neuroscience Research*, *8*, 221–254.

Jastreboff, P. J. (1995). Tinnitus as a phantom perception: Theories and clinical implications. In J. A. Vernon & A. R. Møller (Eds.), *Mechanisms of tinnitus* (pp. 73–93). Needham Heights, MA: Allyn & Bacon.

Jastreboff, P. J. (1996). Clinical implication of the neurophysiological model of tinnitus. In G. E. Reich & J. A. Vernon (Eds.), *Proceedings of the Fifth International Tinnitus Seminar 1995* (pp. 500–507). Portland, OR: American Tinnitus Association.

Jastreboff, P. J. (1998). Tinnitus. In G. A. Gates (Ed.), *Current therapy in otolaryngology-head and neck surgery* (6th ed., pp. 90–95). St. Louis, MO: Mosby-YearBook.

Jastreboff, P. J. (1999a). Categories of the patients in TRT and the treatment outcome. In J. W. P. Hazell (Ed.), *Proceedings of the Sixth International Tinnitus Seminar 1999* (pp. 394–398). London: The Tinnitus and Hyperacusis Centre.

Jastreboff, P. J. (1999b). Optimal sound use in TRT—Theory and practice. In J. Hazell (Ed.), *Proceedings of the Sixth International Tinnitus Seminar 1999* (pp. 491–494). London: The Tinnitus and Hyperacusis Centre.

Jastreboff, P. J. (2000). Tinnitus Habituation Therapy (THT) and Tinnitus Retraining Therapy (TRT). In R. S. Tyler (Ed.), *Tinnitus handbook* (pp. 357–376). San Diego, CA: Singular Publishing Group.

Jastreboff, P. J. (2004). The neurophysiological model of tinnitus. In J. B. Snow (Ed.), *Tinnitus: Theory and management* (pp. 96–107). Lewiston, NY: BC Decker.

Jastreboff, P. J., Gray, W. C., & Gold, S. L. (1996). Neurophysiological approach to tinnitus patients. *The American Journal of Otology*, *17*, 236–240.

Jastreboff, P. J., Hansen, R., Sasaki, P. G., & Sasaki, C. T. (1986). Differential uptake of salicylate in serum, cerebrospinal fluid, and perilymph. *Archives of Otolaryngology-Head and Neck Surgery*, *112*, 1050–1053.

Jastreboff, P. J., & Hazell, J. W. P. (1993). A neurophysiological approach to tinnitus: Clinical implications. *British Journal of Audiology*, *27*, 7–17.

Jastreboff, P. J., & Hazell, J. W. P. (1998). Treatment of tinnitus based on a neurophysiological model. In J. A. Vernon (Ed.), *Tinnitus treatment and relief* (pp. 201–217). Needham Heights, MA: Allyn & Bacon.

Jastreboff, P. J., & Hazell, J. W. P. (2004). *Tinnitus Retraining Therapy: Implementing the neurophysiological model*. New York: Cambridge University Press.

Jastreboff, P. J., Hazell, J. W. P., & Graham, R. L. (1994). Neurophysiological model of tinnitus: Dependence of the minimal masking level on treatment outcome. *Hearing Research*, *80*, 216–232.

Jastreboff, P. J., & Jastreboff, M. M. (1999). How TRT derives from the neurophysiological model. In J. Hazell (Ed.), *Proceedings of the Sixth International*

Tinnitus Seminar 1999 (pp. 87-91). London: The Tinnitus and Hyperacusis Centre.

Jastreboff, P. J., & Jastreboff, M. M. (2000). Tinnitus Retraining Therapy (TRT) as a method for treatment of tinnitus and hyperacusis patients. *Journal of the American Academy of Audiology, 11*, 162-177.

Jastreboff, P. J., & Jastreboff, M. M. (2001). Tinnitus Retraining Therapy. *Seminars in Hearing, 22*, 51-63.

Jastreboff, P. J., & Jastreboff, M. M. (2003). Tinnitus retraining therapy for patients with tinnitus and decreased sound tolerance. *Otolaryngologic Clinics of North America, 36*, 321-336.

Jastreboff, P. J., & Jastreboff, M. M. (2004). Decreased sound tolerance. In J. B. Snow (Ed.), *Tinnitus: Theory and management* (pp. 8-15). Lewiston, NY: BC Decker.

Jastreboff, P. J., & Tarnecki, R. (1975). Response of cat cerebellar vermis induced by sound. II. The role of the mossy and climbing fibers in acoustic transmission to the cerebellar cortex and influence of stimuli parameters. *Acta Neurobiologiae Experimentalis, 35*(3), 217-225.

Johnson, R. M. (1998). The masking of tinnitus. In: J. A. Vernon (Ed.), *Tinnitus treatment and relief* (pp. 164-186). Needham, Mass: Allyn & Bacon.

Jordan, W. P. (1989). Mesencephalic reticular formation lesions made after habituation training abolish long-term habituation of the acoustic startle response in rats. *Behavioral Neuroscience, 103*(4), 805-815.

Jordan, W. P., & Leaton, R. N. (1983). Habituation of the acoustic startle response in rats after lesions in the mesencephalic reticular formation or in the inferior colliculus. *Behavioral Neuroscience, 97*(5), 710-724.

Kaltenbach, J. A. (2000). Neurophysiologic mechanisms of tinnitus. *Journal of the American Academy of Audiology, 11*(3), 125-137.

Kaltenbach, J. A. (2006). The dorsal cochlear nucleus as a participant in the auditory, attentional and emotional components of tinnitus. *Hearing Research, 216-217*, 224-234.

Kaltenbach, J. A., Godfrey, D. A., Neumann, J. B., McCaslin, D. L., Afman, C. E., & Zhang, J. (1998). Changes in spontaneous neural activity in the dorsal cochlear nucleus following exposure to intense sound: Relation to threshold shift. *Hearing Research, 124*(1-2), 78-84.

Kaltenbach, J. A., Zhang, J., & Zacharek, M. A. (2004). Neural correlates of tinnitus. In J. B. Snow (Ed.), *Tinnitus: Theory and management* (pp. 141-161). Lewiston, NY: BC Decker.

Kandel, E. R. (2000a). The brain and behavior. In E. R. Kandel, J. H. Schwartz, & T. M. Jessell (Eds.), *Principles of neural science* (pp. 5-18). New York: McGraw-Hill.

Kandel, E. R. (2000b). Cellular mechanisms of learning and the biological basis of individuality. In E. R. Kandel, J. H. Schwartz, & T. M. Jessell (Eds.), *Principals of neural science* (pp. 1247-1279). New York: McGraw-Hill.

Kandel, E. R. (2000c). From nerve cells to cognition: The internal cellular representation required for perception and action. In E. R. Kandel, J. H. Schwartz, & T. M. Jessell (Eds.), *Principles of neural science* (pp. 381-403). New York: McGraw-Hill.

Kandel, E. R. (2000d). Nerve cells and behavior. In E. R. Kandel, J. H. Schwartz, & T. M. Jessell (Eds.), *Principles of neural science* (pp. 19-35). New York: McGraw-Hill.

Kandel, E. R., Kupfermann, I., & Iversen, S. (2000). Learning and memory. In E. R. Kandel, J. H. Schwartz, & T. M. Jessell (Eds.), *Principles of neural science* (pp. 1227-1246). New York: McGraw-Hill.

Kehoe, E. J., & Macrae, M. (1998). Classical conditioning. In W. O'Donohue (Ed.), *Learning and behavior therapy* (pp. 36-58). Needham Heights, MA: Allyn & Bacon.

Kessels, R. P. (2003). Patients' memory for medical information. *Journal of the Royal Society of Medicine, 96*(5), 219-222.

Kihlstrom, J. F. (1987). The cognitive unconscious. *Science, 237*, 1445-1452.

Kilic, C., Curran, H. V., Noshirvani, H., Marks, I. M., & Basoglu, M. (1999). Long-term effects of alprazolam on memory: A 3.5 year follow-up of agoraphobia/panic patients. *Psychological Medicine, 29*(1), 225-231.

Konorski, J. (1948). *Conditioned reflexes and neuronal organization*. London: Cambridge University Press.

Konorski, J. (1967). *Integrative activity of the brain*. Chicago: University of Chicago Press.

Konorski, J., & Miller, S. (1937). On two types of conditioned reflex. *The Journal of General Psychology, 16*, 264-272.

Kuk, F. K., Tyler, R. S., Russell, D., & Jordan, H. (1990). The psychometric properties of a tinnitus handicap questionnaire. *Ear and Hearing, 11*, 434-445.

Kupfermann, I. (1985). Learning. In E. R. Kandel & J. H. Schwartz (Eds.), *Principles of neural science* (pp. 805-815). New York: Elsevier Science.

Lazarus, A. A. (1971). *Behavior therapy and beyond*. New York: McGraw-Hill.

Lechin, F., van der Dijs, B., & Lechin, M. E. (2002). *Neurocircuitry and neuroautonomic disorders*. Basel, Switzerland: Karger.

LeDoux, J. E. (1992). Emotion and the amygdala. In J. P. Aggleton (Ed.), *The amygdala* (pp. 339-352). New York: Wiley-Liss.

LeDoux, J. E. (1998). *The emotional brain: The mysterious underpinnings of emotional life*. New York: Touchstone.

LeDoux, J. E. (2000). The amygdala and emotion: A view through fear. In J. P. Aggleton (Ed.), *The amygdala: A functional analysis* (pp. 289–310). New York: Oxford University Press.

LeDoux, J. E. (2000). Emotion circuits in the brain. *Annual Review of Neuroscience, 23*, 155–184.

LeDoux, J. E. (2002). *Synaptic self: How our brains become who we are*. New York: Penguin Putnam.

LeDoux, J. E., Farb, C., Ruggiero, D. A., & Reis, D. J. (1987). Thalamus and cortical auditory pathways converge in the rat amygdala. *Society of Neuroscience Abstracts, 13*, 1467.

LeDoux, J. E., Iwata, J., Cicchetti, P., & Reis, D. J. (1988). Different projections of the central amygdaloid nucleus mediate autonomic and behavioral correlates of conditioned fear. *Journal of Neuroscience, 8*, 2517–2529.

Lewicki, P., Hill, T., & Czyzewska, M. (1992). Nonconscious acquisition of information. *American Psychologist, 47*(6), 796–801.

Lindgren, F., & Axelsson, A. (1983). Temporary threshold shift after exposure to noise and music of equal energy. *Ear and Hearing, 4*(4), 197–201.

Lockwood, A. H., Burkard, R. F., & Salvi, R. J. (2004). Imaging tinnitus. In J. B. Snow (Ed.), *Tinnitus: Theory and management* (pp. 253–264). Lewiston, NY: BC Decker.

Lockwood, A. H., Salvi, R. J., Coad, M. L., Towsley, M. L., Wack, D. S., & Murphy, B. W. (1998). The functional neuroanatomy of tinnitus: Evidence for limbic system links and neural plasticity. *Neurology, 50*(1), 114–120.

Lutman, M. E., Brown, E. J., & Coles, R. R. (1987). Self-reported disability and handicap in the population in relation to pure-tone threshold, age, sex and type of hearing loss. *British Journal of Audiology, 21*(1), 45–58.

MacLean, P. D. (1949). Psychosomatic disease and the "visceral brain": Recent developments bearing on the Papez theory of emotion. *Psychosomatic Medicine, 11*, 338-353.

MacLean, P. D. (1952). Some psychiatric implications of physiological studies on fronto-temporal portion of limbic system (visceral brain). *Electroencephalographic Clinical Neurophysiology, 4*, 407–418.

Mahlke, C., & Wallhausser-Franke, E. (2004). Evidence for tinnitus-related plasticity in the auditory and limbic system, demonstrated by arg3.1 and c-fos immunocytochemistry. *Hearing Research, 195*(1–2), 17–34.

Margolis, R. H. (2004). Audiology information counselling—What do patients remember? *Audiology Today, 16*(2), 14–15.

Martinez, J. L., & Derrick, B. E. (1996). Long-term potentiation and learning. *Annual Review of Psychology, 47*, 173–203.

Mathiak, K., Hertrich, I., Grodd, W., & Ackermann, H. (2002). Cerebellum and speech perception: A functional magnetic resonance imaging study. *Journal of Cognitive Neuroscience, 14*(6), 902–912.

McCombe, A., Baguley, D., Coles, R., McKenna, L., McKinney, C., & Windle-Taylor, P. (2001). Guidelines for the grading of tinnitus severity: The results of a working group commissioned by the British Association of Otolaryngologists, Head and Neck Surgeons, 1999. *Clinical Otolaryngology and Allied Sciences, 26*(5), 388–393.

McEwen, B. S., Angulo, J., Cameron, H., Chao, H. M., Daniels, D., Gannon, M. N., et al. (1992). Paradoxical effects of adrenal steroids on the brain: Protection versus degeneration. *Biological Psychiatry, 31*(2), 177–199.

McKenna, L. (2004). Models of tinnitus suffering and treatment compared and contrasted. *Audiological Medicine, 2*, 41–53.

McKinney, C. J., Hazell, J. W. P., & Graham, R. L. (1999). Changes in loudness discomfort level and sensitivity to environmental sound with habituation based therapy. In J. Hazell (Ed.), *Proceedings of the Sixth International Tinnitus Seminar* (pp. 499–501). London: The Tinnitus and Hyperacusis Centre.

Meikle, M. B. (1991a). How tinnitus is related to hearing impairment. In *Assessment and Re-Habilitation: Papers presented at 3rd Bi-Annual Workshop, 15th–17th March 1991* (pp. 4–6). Melbourne: Australian Association of Audiologists in Private Practice.

Meikle, M. B. (1991b). Methods for evaluation of tinnitus relief procedures. In J.-M. Aran & R. Dauman (Eds.), *Proceedings IV International Tinnitus Seminar, Bordeaux* (pp. 555–562). New York: Kugler.

Meikle, M. B., Abrams, H. B., Newman, C. W., Sandridge, S. A., & Henry, J. A. (2005). Empirical development of a new tinnitus outcome measure. *American Auditory Society Bulletin, 30*, 26.

Meikle, M. B., Creedon, T. A., Abrams, H. B., Henry, J. A., Newman, C. W., & Sandridge, S. (2005). An innovative method for developing a new tinnitus outcome questionnaire: Use of a Web-based intranet to solicit expert decisions concerning content validity. *Abstracts of the Association of Research in Otolaryngology, 28*, 61.

Meikle, M. B., Creedon, T. A., & Griest, S. E. (2004). *Tinnitus archive 2d ed.* Retrieved April 29, 2004, from http://www.tinnitusarchive.org

Meikle, M. B., & Griest, S. E. (1989). Gender-based differences in characteristics of tinnitus. *The Hearing Journal, 42*, 68–76.

Meikle, M. B., & Griest, S. E. (2002). Tinnitus severity and disability: Prospective efforts to develop a core set of measures. In R. Patuzzi (Ed.), *VIIth International Tinnitus Seminar* (pp. 157-161). Perth: Physiology Dept., Univ. of Western Australia.

Meikle, M. B., Vernon, J., & Johnson, R. M. (1984). The perceived severity of tinnitus. *Otolaryngology-Head and Neck Surgery*, *92*(6), 689-696.

Mencher, G. T., Gerber, S. E., & McCombe, A. (1997). *Audiology and auditory dysfunction*. Needham Heights, MA: Allyn & Bacon.

Miller, G. A. (1956). The magical number seven plus or minus two: Some limits on our capacity for processing information. *Psychological Review*, *63*(2), 81-97.

Mineka, S., & Hamida, S. B. (1998). Observational and nonconscious learning. In W. O'Donohue (Ed.), *Learning and behavior therapy* (pp. 421-439). Needham Heights, MA: Allyn & Bacon.

Møller, A. R. (2003). Pathophysiology of tinnitus. *Otolaryngologic Clinics of North America*, *36*(2), 249-266, v-vi.

National Center for PTSD. (2005). Department of Veterans Affairs, National Center for PTSD.

National Institutes of Health Consensus. (1994). Development conference statement on acoustic neuroma. *Archives of Neurology*, *51*, 201-207.

Newman, C. W., Jacobson, G. P., & Spitzer, J. B. (1996). Development of the Tinnitus Handicap Inventory. *Archives of Otolaryngology-Head and Neck Surgery*, *122*, 143-148.

Newman, C. W., & Sandridge, S. A. (2004). Tinnitus questionnaires. In J. B. Snow (Ed.), *Tinnitus: Theory and management* (pp. 237-254). Lewiston, NY: BC Decker.

Newman, C. W., Sandridge, S. A., & Jacobson, G. P. (1998). Psychometric adequacy of the Tinnitus Handicap Inventory (THI) for evaluating treatment outcome. *Journal of the American Academy of Audiology*, *9*, 153-160.

NIDCD. Noise-induced hearing loss. (2004). Bethesda, MD: National Institute of Deafness and Other Communicative Disorders (NIDCD). Retrieved January 29, 2007, from http://www.nidcd.nih.gov/health/hearing/noise.asp#who

Oertel, D., & Young, E. D. (2004). What's a cerebellar circuit doing in the auditory system? *Trends in Neuroscience*, *27*(2), 104-110.

Pavlov, I. P. (1927). *Conditioned reflexes*. Oxford: Oxford University Press.

Pearson, J. D., Morrell, C. H., Gordon-Salant, S., Brant, L. J., Metter, E. J., Klein, L. L., et al. (1995). Gender differences in a longitudinal study of age-associated hearing loss. *Journal of the Acoustical Society of America*, *97*(2), 1196-1205.

Penner, M. J. (1983). Variability in matches to subjective tinnitus. *Journal of Speech and Hearing Research*, *26*, 263-267.

Penner, M. J., Brauth, S., & Hood, L. (1981). The temporal course of the masking of tinnitus as a basis for inferring its origin. *Journal of Speech and Hearing Research*, *24*, 257-261.

Perry, B. P., & Gantz, B. J. (2000). Medical and surgical evaluation and management of tinnitus. In R. S. Tyler (Ed.), *Tinnitus handbook* (pp. 221-241). San Diego, CA: Singular Publishing Group.

Petrides, M. (1994). Frontal lobes and behaviour. *Current Opinions in Neurobiology*, *4*(2), 207-211.

Pitkanen, A. (2000). Connectivity of the rat amygdaloid complex. In J. P. Aggleton (Ed.), *The amygdala: A functional analysis* (pp. 31-115). New York: Oxford University Press Inc.

Posner, M. I., & Driver, J. (1992). The neurobiology of selective attention. *Current Opinions in Neurobiology*, *2*(2), 165-169.

Pribram, K. H. (1987). Holography and brain function. In G. Adelman (Ed.), *Encyclopedia of neuroscience* (pp. 499-500). Boston: Birkhauser.

Punch, J., Joseph, A., & Rakerd, B. (2004). Most comfortable and uncomfortable loudness levels: Six decades of research. *American Journal of Audiology*, *13*, 144-157.

Reber, A. S. (1989). Implicit learning and tacit knowledge. *Journal of Experimental Psychology: General*, *118*, 219-235.

Reed, G. F. (1960). An audiometric study of two hundred cases of subjective tinnitus. *Archives of Otolaryngology*, *71*, 94-104.

Reyes, S. A., Salvi, R. J., Burkard, R. F., Coad, M. L., Wack, D. S., Galantowicz, P. J., et al. (2002). Brain imaging of the effects of lidocaine on tinnitus. *Hearing Research*, *171*(1-2), 43-50.

Rice, C. G. (1994). Annoyance due to low frequency hums. *British Medical Journal*, *308*(6925), 355-356.

Robinson, S. K., Viirre, E. S., & Stein, M. B. (2004). Antidepressant therapy for tinnitus. In J. B. Snow (Ed.), *Tinnitus: Theory and management* (pp. 278-293). Lewiston, NY: BC Decker.

Saper, C. B. (2000a). Brain stem modulation of sensation, movement, and consciousness. In E. R. Kandel, J. H. Schwartz, & T. M. Jessell (Eds.), *Principles of neural science* (pp. 889-909). New York: McGraw-Hill.

Saper, C. B. (2000b). Brain stem, reflexive behavior, and the cranial nerves. In E. R. Kandel, J. H. Schwartz, & T. M. Jessell (Eds.), *Principles of neural science* (pp. 873-888). New York: McGraw-Hill.

Schechter, M. A., & Henry, J. A. (2002). Assessment and treatment of tinnitus patients using a "masking approach." *Journal of the American Academy of Audiology*, *13*, 545–558.

Scott, B., Lindberg, P., Melin, L., & Lyttkens, L. (1990). Predictors of tinnitus discomfort, adaptation and subjective loudness. *British Journal of Audiology*, *24*, 51–62.

Searchfield, G. D. (2005). Hearing aids and tinnitus. In R. S. Tyler (Ed.), *Tinnitus treatment: Clinical protocols* (pp. 161–175). New York: Thieme.

Shapiro, D. E., Boggs, S. R., Melamed, B. G., & Graham-Pole, J. (1992). The effect of varied physician affect on recall, anxiety, and perceptions in women at risk for breast cancer: An analogue study. *Health Psychology*, *11*(1), 61–66.

Sheldrake, J. B., Jastreboff, P. J., & Hazell, J. W. P. (1996). Perspectives for total elimination of tinnitus perception. In G. E. Reich & J. A. Vernon (Eds.), *Proceedings of the Fifth International Tinnitus Seminar 1995* (pp. 531–536). Portland, OR: American Tinnitus Association.

Shore, S. E. (2004). Sensory nuclei in tinnitus. In J. B. Snow (Ed.), *Tinnitus: Theory and management* (pp. 125–139). Lewiston, NY: BC Decker.

Sismanis, A. (1998). Pulsatile tinnitus. In J. A. Vernon (Ed.), *Tinnitus treatment and relief* (pp. 28–33). Needham Heights, MA: Allyn & Bacon.

Skinner, B. F. (1953). *Science and human behavior*. New York: Free Press.

Skinner, M. W. (1988). *Hearing aid evaluation*. Englewood Cliffs, NJ: Prentice Hall.

Spielberger, C. D. (1983). *State-trait anxiety inventory for adults*. Palo Alto, CA: Mind Garden.

Stewart, M., Brown, J. B., Donner, A., McWhinney, I. R., Oates, J., Weston, W. W., et al. (2000). The impact of patient-centered care on outcomes. *Journal of Family Practice*, *49*, 796–804.

Swanson, S. J., Dengerink, H. A., Kondrick, P., & Miller, C. L. (1987). The influence of subjective factors on temporary threshold shifts after exposure to music and noise of equal energy. *Ear and Hearing*, *8*(5), 288–291.

Thompson, R. F. (1967). *Foundations of physiological psychology*. New York: Harper & Row.

Thompson, R. F., & Donegan, N. H. (1987). Learning and memory. In G. Adelman (Ed.), *Encyclopedia of neuroscience* (Vol. 1, pp. 571–574). Boston: Birkhauser.

Tonndorf, J. (1995). The analogy between tinnitus and pain: A suggestion for a physiological basis of chronic tinnitus. In J. A. Vernon & A. R. Møller (Eds.), *Mechanisms of tinnitus* (pp. 231–235). Needham Heights, MA: Allyn & Bacon.

Tyler, R. S. (1993). Tinnitus disability and handicap questionnaires. *Seminars in Hearing*, *14*, 377–383.

Tyler, R. S. (Ed.). (2005). *Tinnitus treatment: Clinical protocols*. New York: Thieme.

Tyler, R. S., & Baker, L. J. (1983). Difficulties experienced by tinnitus sufferers. *Journal of Speech and Hearing Disorders*, *48*, 150–154.

Tyler, R. S., & Conrad-Armes, D. (1983). Tinnitus pitch: A comparison of three measurement methods. *British Journal of Audiology*, *17*, 101–107.

Tyler, R. S., Noble, W., Preece, J. P., Dunn, C. C., & Witt, S. A. (2004). Psychological treatments for tinnitus. In J. B. Snow (Ed.), *Tinnitus: Theory and management* (pp. 314–323). Lewiston, NY: BC Decker.

Uylings, H. B., & van Eden, C. G. (1990). Qualitative and quantitative comparison of the prefrontal cortex in rat and in primates, including humans. *Progressive Brain Research*, *85*, 31–62.

Vander, A. J., Sherman, J. H., & Luciano, D. S. (1990). *Human physiology* (5th ed.). New York: McGraw-Hill.

Vernon, J. A. (1976). The loudness (?) of tinnitus. *Hearing and Speech Action*, *44*, 17–19.

Vernon, J. A. (1992). Tinnitus: Causes, evaluation, and treatment. In G. M. English (Ed.), *Otolaryngology* (Rev. ed., pp. 1–25). Philadelphia: JB Lippincott.

Vernon, J. A. (1998). *Tinnitus treatment and relief*. Needham Heights, MA: Allyn & Bacon.

Vernon, J. A. (2002). Hyperacusis: Testing, treatments and a possible mechanism. *The Australian and New Zealand Journal of Audiology*, *24*, 68–73.

Vernon, J. A., & Fenwick, J. (1984). Identification of tinnitus: A plea for standardization. *Journal of Laryngology and Otology*, *S9:45*, 45–53.

Vernon, J. A., & Meikle, M. B. (1981). Tinnitus masking: Unresolved problems. In D. Evered & G. Lawrenson (Eds.), *Ciba Foundation Symposium 85. Tinnitus* (pp. 239–256). London: Pitman Books.

Vernon, J. A., & Meikle, M. B. (1988). Measurement of tinnitus: An update. In M. Kitahara (Ed.), *Tinnitus. Pathophysiology and Management* (pp. 36–52). Tokyo: Igaku-Shoin.

Vernon, J. A., & Meikle, M. B. (2000). Tinnitus masking. In R. S. Tyler (Ed.), *Tinnitus handbook* (pp. 313–356). San Diego: Singular Publishing Group.

Vernon, J. A., & Meikle, M. B. (2003). Tinnitus: Clinical measurement. *The Otolaryngologic Clinics of North America*, *36*(2), 293–305, vi.

Vernon, J. A., & Press, L. (1998). Treatment for hyperacusis. In J. A. Vernon (Ed.), *Tinnitus treatment and relief* (pp. 223–227). Needham Heights, MA: Allyn & Bacon.

Verwey, B., Eling, P., Wientjes, H., & Zitman, F. G. (2000). Memory impairment in those who attempted suicide by benzodiazepine overdose. *Journal of Clinical Psychiatry, 61*(6), 456–459; quiz 460.

Victor, M., & Ropper, A. H. (2001). *Adams and Victor's principles of neurology* (7th ed.). New York: McGraw-Hill.

Wackym, P. A., & Friedland, D. R. (2004). Otologic evaluation. In J. B. Snow (Ed.), *Tinnitus: Theory and management* (pp. 205–219). Lewiston, NY: BC Decker.

Wallhausser-Franke, E., Mahlke, C., Oliva, R., Braun, S., Wenz, G., & Langner, G. (2003). Expression of c-fos in auditory and non-auditory brain regions of the gerbil after manipulations that induce tinnitus. *Experimental Brain Research, 153*(4), 649–654.

Weiss, S. R. B., Li, H., Sitcoske-O'Shea, M., & Post, R.M. (2000). Amygdala plasticity: The neurobiological implications of kindling. In J. P. Aggleton (Ed.), *The amygdala: A functional analysis* (pp. 155–194). New York: Oxford University Press.

Westbrook, G. L. (2000). Seizures and epilepsy. In E. R. Kandel. J. H. Schwartz, & T. M. Jessell (Eds.), *Principles of neural science* (pp. 910–935). New York: McGraw-Hill.

Wilson, P. H. (2006). Classical conditioning as the basis for the effective treatment of tinnitus-related distress. *ORL; Journal for Oto-Rhino-Laryngology and Its Related Specialties 68*(1), 6–11; discussion 11–13.

Wilson, P. H., Henry, J. L., Andersson, G., Hallam, R. S., & Lindberg, P. (1998). A critical analysis of directive counselling as a component of tinnitus retraining therapy. *British Journal of Audiology, 32*, 273–287.

Wilson-Pauwels, L., Stewart, P. A., & Akesson, E. J. (1997). *Autonomic nerves*. Hamilton, Ontario: BC Decker.

Wolk, C., & Seefeld, B. (1999). The effects of managing hyperacusis with maskers (noise generators). In J. Hazell (Ed.), *Proceedings of the Sixth International Tinnitus Seminar* (pp. 512–514). London: The Tinnitus and Hyperacusis Centre.

Woody, C. D., Wang, X. F., & Gruen, W. E. (1998). Acoustic transmission in the dentate nucleus. I. Patterns of activity to click and hiss; II. Changes in activity and excitability after conditioning. *Brain Research, 789*(1), 74–83.

Zaugg, T., Schechter, M. A., Fausti, S. A., & Henry, J. A. (2002). Difficulties caused by patients' misconceptions that hearing problems are due to tinnitus. In R. Patuzzi (Ed.), *Proceedings of the Seventh International Tinnitus Seminar* (pp. 226–228). Crawley: The University of Western Australia.

Zhang, J. S., Kaltenbach, J. A., Wang, J., & Kim, S. A. (2003). Fos-like immunoreactivity in auditory and nonauditory brain structures of hamsters previously exposed to intense sound. *Experimental Brain Research, 153*(4), 655–660.

Ziemann, U., Hallett, M., & Cohen, L. G. (1998). Mechanisms of deafferentation-induced plasticity in human motor cortex. *Journal of Neuroscience, 18*(17), 7000–7007.

APPENDIX A

TRT Initial Interview

Patient ID#: ______________________ Visit #______________________ Date: ______________________

*Before I ask these questions, I need to explain that we are evaluating three different things: (1) tinnitus, (2) sound tolerance, and (3) hearing. Each question is specific to **tinnitus**, **sound tolerance**, or **hearing. Tinnitus** refers to any kind of sound in your head—ringing, hissing, and so on. **Sound tolerance** refers to how you react to different sounds around you. **Hearing** refers to your ability to detect sounds around you, or to your ability to understand the speech of others. Before we go on, is it clear how these differ?*

*The questions about your tinnitus generally refer to the **last month**. Answer these questions thinking about your tinnitus **over the last month**. I also need to tell you that some of these questions may seem repetitive or redundant to you. However, I need all of the answers to come directly from you, even if I may already know the answer. Also, please know that there are **no wrong answers**.*

TINNITUS

*The first series of questions are specific to your **tinnitus**. Please think only about your **tinnitus** when you answer these questions.*

1. What does your **most bothersome** tinnitus sound like? (check **one box only**)

☐ Ringing
☐ Hissing
☐ Clear tone
☐ High-tension wire
☐ Buzzing
☐ More than 1 tone
☐ Crickets
☐ Whistle
☐ Hum
☐ Pulsating
☐ Ocean Roar
☐ Pounding
☐ Music
☐ Transformer noise
☐ Clicking
☐ Sizzling
☐ Other sound ______________________

2. Where is the location of your **most bothersome** tinnitus? (check **one box only**)

☐ Right ear only
☐ Left ear only
☐ Both ears
☐ Not sure
☐ Inside of head
☐ Outside of head
☐ Other ______________________

3. Is your tinnitus louder on one side of your head than the other?

☐ Right louder than left
☐ Left louder than right
☐ Equal

4. Is your tinnitus a constant sound or an intermittent sound?

- ☐ Constant
- ☐ Intermittent

5. Does the loudness of your tinnitus change on its own?

- ☐ No—**Go to Question 6**
- ☐ Yes—How often does it change?
  - ☐ Never
  - ☐ Several times per month
  - ☐ Several times per week
  - ☐ Several times per day
  - ☐ Several times per hour

(Interviewer: If female respondent, ask if fluctuation in tinnitus volume is related to menstrual cycle—select N/A if subject is male)

- ☐ No
- ☐ Yes
- ☐ N/A

6. Please describe the onset of your tinnitus:

- ☐ Gradual
- ☐ Sudden

How long have you had your tinnitus?

☐ Less than 1 year	☐ 6–10 years
☐ 1–2 years	☐ 11–20 years
☐ 3–5 years	☐ More than 20 years

7. Do you have "bad days" when your tinnitus is more bothersome than usual, or does it seem equally bothersome from day to day?

- ☐ No, doesn't have "bad days"—**Go to Question 8**
- ☐ Yes, has "bad days"—How often do you have these "bad days?"

☐ 1	*days per*	☐ Week
☐ 2		☐ Month
☐ 3		☐ Year
☐ 4		
☐ 5 or more		

8. Do sounds ever cause a change in the loudness of your tinnitus?

- ☐ No effect—**Go to Question 9**
- ☐ Softer—**Go to Question 9**
- ☐ Louder

(If LOUDER) What kinds of sounds cause this change? **(Interviewer:** Ask as an open-ended question; do not read list to patient; check all categories that apply)

- ☐ **Very loud sounds/activities** that would be expected to cause a change in the loudness of tinnitus (e.g., firing a gun, attending a concert, using power tools)
- ☐ **Higher pitched sounds** (e.g., squeals, squeaks, beeps, whistles, rings)
- ☐ **Lower pitched sounds** (e.g., bass from radio)

☐ **Traffic (warning) sounds** (e.g., emergency vehicle sirens, car horns, back-up beeper on truck/van)
☐ **Traffic (background) sounds** (e.g., road noise, road construction, diesel engines, garbage trucks)
☐ **Sudden impact sounds** (e.g., door slam, car backfiring, objects dropping on floor, dishes clattering)
☐ **Voices** (e.g., television, radio, movies, children's voices, dog barking)
☐ **Other** (describe) ______________________________

When any of these sounds cause your tinnitus to change, how long does the change last?

☐ 1–2	☐ Seconds
☐ 3–4	☐ Minutes
☐ 5–10	☐ Hours
☐ more than 10	☐ Days

When you hear a sound that causes your tinnitus to change, does the effect sometimes last until the next morning after you've slept?
☐ No—**Go to Question 9**
☐ Yes

(If EFFECT LASTS AT LEAST UNTIL THE NEXT MORNING) What kinds of sounds cause this to happen? (**Interviewer:** Ask as an open-ended question; do not read list to patient; check all categories that apply)
☐ **Very loud sounds/activities** (e.g., firing a gun, attending a concert, using power tools)
☐ **Higher pitched sounds** (e.g., squeals, squeaks, beeps, whistles, rings)
☐ **Lower pitched sounds** (e.g., bass from radio)
☐ **Traffic (warning) sounds** (e.g., emergency vehicle sirens, car horns, back-up beeper on truck/van)
☐ **Traffic (background) sounds** (e g., road noise, road construction, diesel engines, garbage trucks)
☐ **Sudden impact sounds** (e.g., door slam, car backfiring, objects dropping on floor, dishes clattering)
☐ **Voices** (e.g., television, radio, movies, children's voices, dog barking)
☐ **Other** (describe) ______________________________

9. Do you use ear protection (earplugs or earmuffs)?
☐ No—**Go to Question 10**
☐ Yes

(If YES) Why do you use ear protection?
☐ To keep tinnitus from getting louder
☐ Trouble tolerating everyday sounds that seem normal to others
☐ Other ______________________________

(**Interviewer:** Determine if the patient uses ear protection specifically because of tinnitus—this would usually be to prevent the tinnitus from getting louder, which should not be suggested to the patient to avoid "negative counseling." Also, determine if the patient uses ear protection specifically because of trouble tolerating environmental sounds that seem normal to others—this too should not be suggested to avoid negative counseling. Other reasons for using ear protection do not need to be recorded.)

If EAR PROTECTION IS USED FOR TINNITUS: What percent of the time do you use earplugs or earmuffs **for your tinnitus**?

☐ 5%	☐ 30%	☐ 55%	☐ 80%
☐ 10%	☐ 35%	☐ 60%	☐ 85%
☐ 15%	☐ 40%	☐ 65%	☐ 90%
☐ 20%	☐ 45%	☐ 70%	☐ 95%
☐ 25%	☐ 50%	☐ 75%	☐ 100%

Do you use your earplugs or earmuffs **for your tinnitus** when it's fairly quiet?

☐ No
☐ Yes

Interviewer: Does patient **overprotect** ears because of tinnitus? (if so, discuss importance of not overprotecting)

☐ No
☐ Yes

10. Are you currently receiving any other treatment specifically for your tinnitus?

☐ No—**Go to Question 11**
☐ Yes

(If YES) What?

☐ Herbs	☐ Counseling
☐ Vitamins	☐ Tabletop sound machines
☐ Hypnosis	☐ Special CDs or tapes
☐ Acupuncture	☐ Other ________________

11. What is the **biggest reason** your tinnitus is a problem (not including trouble hearing or trouble understanding speech)? ____

12. I'm going to read through a list of activities and I want you to tell me how often your tinnitus keeps you from doing these activities, or how often it negatively affects these activities in any way. Please don't include trouble hearing or trouble understanding speech when you answer these questions.

	Never	Rarely	Sometimes	Often	Always	N/A
a. Concentration?	☐	☐	☐	☐	☐	☐
b. Sleep?	☐	☐	☐	☐	☐	☐
c. Quiet resting activities (reading, relaxing, etc.)?	☐	☐	☐	☐	☐	☐

(**Interviewer:** For questions d through i, if the patient reports an effect from tinnitus, ask the patient **how** or **why** the activity is affected. You do not need to record how or why the activity is affected—this is asked to ensure that the patient is not including hearing difficulties in the responses.)

	Never	Rarely	Sometimes	Often	Always	N/A
d. Work? (select N/A if retired)	☐	☐	☐	☐	☐	☐
e. Day-to-day responsibilities outside of work?	☐	☐	☐	☐	☐	☐
f. Going to restaurants?	☐	☐	☐	☐	☐	☐
g. Participating in or observing sports events?	☐	☐	☐	☐	☐	☐

	Never	Rarely	Sometimes	Often	Always	N/A
h. Social activities?	☐	☐	☐	☐	☐	☐
i. Anything else? ______________	☐	☐	☐	☐	☐	☐

13. What percent of your **total awake time**, over the last month, were you **noticing, or thinking about**, your tinnitus? Please give an average percentage over the last month.

☐ 5%	☐ 30%	☐ 55%	☐ 80%
☐ 10%	☐ 35%	☐ 60%	☐ 85%
☐ 15%	☐ 40%	☐ 65%	☐ 90%
☐ 20%	☐ 45%	☐ 70%	☐ 95%
☐ 25%	☐ 50%	☐ 75%	☐ 100%

14. What percent of your **total awake time**, over the last month, were you **annoyed, distressed, or irritated** by your tinnitus? Please give an average percentage over the last month.

☐ 5%	☐ 30%	☐ 55%	☐ 80%
☐ 10%	☐ 35%	☐ 60%	☐ 85%
☐ 15%	☐ 40%	☐ 65%	☐ 90%
☐ 20%	☐ 45%	☐ 70%	☐ 95%
☐ 25%	☐ 50%	☐ 75%	☐ 100%

(**Interviewer**: Double-check that patient responded appropriately to Questions 13 and 14, i.e., to **total awake time for each condition of awareness and annoyance**)

I'm now going to ask you to rank your tinnitus, on a scale of 0 to 10, with regard to severity, annoyance, and effect on your life. Please do not include trouble hearing or trouble understanding speech when you answer these questions.

15. How **strong**, or **loud**, was your tinnitus, on average, over the last month? "0" would be "no tinnitus"; "10" would be "as loud as you can imagine."

(no tinnitus) **0 1 2 3 4 5 6 7 8 9 10** **(as loud as imaginable)**

16. How much has tinnitus **annoyed you**, on average, over the last month—not including annoyance from trouble hearing or trouble understanding speech? "0" would be "not annoying at all"; "10" would be "as annoying as you can imagine."

(not annoying) **0 1 2 3 4 5 6 7 8 9 10** **(as annoying as imaginable)**

17. How much did tinnitus **impact your life**, on average, over the last month—not including impact from trouble hearing or trouble understanding speech? "0" would be "not at all"; "10" would be "as much as you can imagine."

(no impact) **0 1 2 3 4 5 6 7 8 9 10** **(as much impact as imaginable)**

18. Do you have any other comments about your tinnitus? ______________________________

SOUND TOLERANCE

The next series of questions is only about your ***ability to tolerate sound****. Please think only about* ***sound tolerance*** *when you answer these questions.*

19. Are sounds bothersome or unpleasant to you when they seem normal to other people around you?
- ☐ No—**Go to Question 31**
- ☐ Yes

(If YES) What kinds of sounds are bothersome or unpleasant? **(Interviewer:** Ask as an open-ended question; do not read list to patient; check all categories that apply)
- ☐ **Higher pitched sounds** (e.g., squeals, squeaks, beeps, whistles, rings)
- ☐ **Lower pitched sounds** (e.g., bass from radio, next door music)
- ☐ **Traffic (warning) sounds** (e.g., emergency vehicle sirens, car horns, back-up beeper on truck/van)
- ☐ **Traffic (background) sounds** (e.g., road noise, road construction, diesel engines, garbage trucks)
- ☐ **Sudden impact sounds** (e.g., door slam, car backfiring, objects dropping on floor, dishes clattering)
- ☐ **Voices** (e.g., television, radio, movies, children's voices, dog barking)
- ☐ **Other** (describe) ______________________________

20. Do these sounds cause you pain or physical discomfort?
- ☐ No
- ☐ Yes

21. Do you have "bad days" when sound tolerance is more of a problem than on other days, or is your ability to tolerate sound the same from day to day?
- ☐ No, doesn't have "bad days"—**Go to Question 22**
- ☐ Yes, has "bad days"—How often do you have these "bad days?"

☐ 1	*days per*	☐ Week
☐ 2		☐ Month
☐ 3		☐ Year
☐ 4		
☐ 5 or more		

22. Do sounds ever cause a change in how much sound you can tolerate?
- ☐ No effect—**Go to Question 23**
- ☐ Better able to tolerate sound—**Go to Question 23**
- ☐ Less able to tolerate sound

(If LESS ABLE TO TOLERATE SOUND) What kinds of sounds have this effect? **(Interviewer:** Ask as an open-ended question; do not read list to patient; check all categories that apply)
- ☐ **Very loud sounds/activities** (e.g., firing a gun, attending a concert, using power tools)
- ☐ **Higher pitched sounds** (e.g., squeals, squeaks, beeps, whistles, rings)
- ☐ **Lower pitched sounds** (e.g., bass from radio)
- ☐ **Traffic (warning) sounds** (e.g., emergency vehicle sirens, car horns, back-up beeper on truck/van)
- ☐ **Traffic (background) sounds** (e.g., road noise, road construction, diesel engines, garbage trucks)

☐ **Sudden impact sounds** (e.g., door slam, car backfiring, objects dropping on floor, dishes clattering)
☐ **Voices** (e.g., television, radio, movies, children's voices, dog barking)
☐ **Other** (describe) ______________________________

When any of these sounds reduce your sound tolerance, how long does the change last?

☐ 1–2	☐ Seconds
☐ 3–4	☐ Minutes
☐ 5–10	☐ Hours
☐ more than 10	☐ Days

When you hear a sound that reduces your ability to tolerate sounds, does the effect sometimes last until the next morning after you've slept?
☐ No—**Go to Question 23**
☐ Yes

(If EFFECT LASTS AT LEAST UNTIL NEXT MORNING) What kinds of sounds cause this to happen? **(Interviewer:** Ask as an open-ended question; do not read list to patient; check all categories that apply)
☐ **Very loud sounds/activities** (e.g., firing a gun, attending a concert, using power tools)
☐ **Higher pitched sounds** (e.g., squeals, squeaks, beeps, whistles, rings)
☐ **Lower pitched sounds** (e.g., bass from radio)
☐ **Traffic (warning) sounds** (e.g., emergency vehicle sirens, car horns, back-up beeper on truck/van)
☐ **Traffic (background) sounds** (e.g., road noise, road construction, diesel engines, garbage trucks)
☐ **Sudden impact sounds** (e.g., door slam, car backfiring, objects dropping on floor, dishes clattering)
☐ **Voices** (e.g., television, radio, movies, children's voices, dog barking)
☐ **Other** (describe) ______________________________

23. **(Interviewer:** In Question 9 did the patient report the use of hearing protection because of "trouble tolerating everyday sounds"?)
☐ No—**Go to Question 24**
☐ Yes

(If YES) Earlier you told me that you sometimes use ear protection because of trouble tolerating sound—what percent of the time do you use ear protection **because of that trouble**?

☐ 5%	☐ 30%	☐ 55%	☐ 80%
☐ 10%	☐ 35%	☐ 60%	☐ 85%
☐ 15%	☐ 40%	☐ 65%	☐ 90%
☐ 20%	☐ 45%	☐ 70%	☐ 95%
☐ 25%	☐ 50%	☐ 75%	☐ 100%

(If YES) Do you use your earplugs when it's fairly quiet **because of trouble tolerating sound**?
☐ No
☐ Yes

(Interviewer: does patient **overprotect** ears **due to problems with sound tolerance**?)
☐ No
☐ Yes

24. Are you currently receiving any treatment specifically for problems with **sound tolerance**?

☐ No—**Go to Question 25**
☐ Yes

(If YES) What?

☐ Herbs	☐ Counseling
☐ Vitamins	☐ Tabletop sound machines
☐ Hypnosis	☐ Special CDs or tapes
☐ Acupuncture	☐ Other ________________

25. What is the major reason **trouble tolerating sound** is a problem?

____

26. I'm going to read a list of activities and I want you to tell me how often trouble tolerating sound keeps you from doing these activities, or how often it negatively affects these activities in any way.

	Never	Rarely	Sometimes	Often	Always	N/A
a. Concerts?	☐	☐	☐	☐	☐	☐
b. Shopping?	☐	☐	☐	☐	☐	☐
c. Movies?	☐	☐	☐	☐	☐	☐
d. Work? (select N/A if retired)	☐	☐	☐	☐	☐	☐
e. Day-to-day responsibilities outside of work?	☐	☐	☐	☐	☐	☐
f. Going to restaurants?	☐	☐	☐	☐	☐	☐
g. Driving?	☐	☐	☐	☐	☐	☐
h. Participating in or observing sports events?	☐	☐	☐	☐	☐	☐
i. Attending church?	☐	☐	☐	☐	☐	☐
j. Housekeeping activities?	☐	☐	☐	☐	☐	☐
k. Child care?	☐	☐	☐	☐	☐	☐
l. Social activities?	☐	☐	☐	☐	☐	☐
m. Anything else? ________________	☐	☐	☐	☐	☐	☐

*I'm now going to ask you to rank your **sound tolerance**, on a scale of 0 to 10, with regard to severity, annoyance, and effect on your life.*

27. Please rate your **ability to tolerate sound** on a scale of "0" to "10." "0" would mean "you can tolerate all sounds"; "10" would mean "you cannot tolerate any sounds."

(can tolerate all) **0 1 2 3 4 5 6 7 8 9 10** **(cannot tolerate any)**

28. How much has trouble tolerating sound **annoyed you,** on average, over the last month? "0" would be "not annoying at all"; "10" would be "as annoying as you can imagine."

(not annoying) **0 1 2 3 4 5 6 7 8 9 10** **(as annoying as imaginable)**

29. How much did trouble tolerating sound **affect your life**, on average, over the last month? "0" would be "not at all"; "10" would be "as much as you can imagine."

(not at all) **0 1 2 3 4 5 6 7 8 9 10** **(as much as imaginable)**

30. Do you have any other comments about **trouble tolerating sound**?

____

HEARING

I now have just a few questions about your hearing ability.

31. Do you think you have a hearing problem?
- ☐ No
- ☐ Yes
- ☐ Not sure

32. Have you ever worn hearing aids?
- ☐ No
- ☐ Yes

33. Has anyone ever suggested that you try hearing aids?
- ☐ No—**Go to Question 34**
- ☐ Yes

(If YES) From whom?
- ☐ A professional
- ☐ Family
- ☐ Friend
- ☐ Other ____________________

RANKING PROBLEMS

Next, I'm going to ask you to rank how much of a problem tinnitus, sound tolerance, and hearing were ***on average over the last month*** *on a scale of 1 to 10.* (**Interviewer**: Do not ask patient about sound tolerance or hearing if they were not identified as a problem—circle "0" in that instance.)

34. How much of a problem is **tinnitus** (if you are not including problems from trouble hearing or trouble understanding speech)? "0" would be "no problem at all"; "10" would be "as much as you can imagine."

(no problem) 0 1 2 3 4 5 6 7 8 9 10 **(as much as imaginable)**

35. How much of a problem is **trouble tolerating sound**? "0" would be "no problem at all"; "10" would be "as much as you can imagine."

(no problem) 0 1 2 3 4 5 6 7 8 9 10 **(as much as imaginable)**

36. How much of a problem is **hearing**? "0" would be "no problem at all"; "10" would be "as much as you can imagine."

(no problem) 0 1 2 3 4 5 6 7 8 9 10 **(as much as imaginable)**

Interviewer:

(A) Indicate patient TRT **category**:

- ☐ Category 0
- ☐ Category 1
- ☐ Category 2
- ☐ Category 3
- ☐ Category 4

(B) Recommendation: ______________________________

(C) Patient decision: ______________________________

(D) Next visit: ______________________________

Portions of this form adapted from Henry, J. A., Jastreboff, M. M., Jastreboff, P. J., Schechter, M. A., & Fausti, S. A. (2003); Henry, J A., Zaugg, T. L., & Schechter, M. A., (2005); Johnson (1998); and Jastreboff, P. J. & Hazell, J. W. P. (2004). Adapted with permission from the authors.

APPENDIX B

TRT Follow-Up Interview

Patient ID#: ____________________ Visit #____________________ Date: ____________________

*These questions are basically the same as the questions you were asked at your initial evaluation. Recall that we are evaluating three different things: (1) tinnitus, (2) sound tolerance, and (3) hearing. Each question is specific to **tinnitus**, **sound tolerance**, or **hearing**. **Tinnitus** refers to any kind of sound in your head—ringing, hissing, and so on. **Sound tolerance** refers to how you react to different sounds around you. **Hearing** refers to your ability to detect sounds around you, or to your ability to understand the speech of others. Before we go on, are these definitions clear?*

*The questions about your tinnitus generally refer to the **last month**. Answer these questions thinking about your tinnitus **over the last month**. These questions may seem repetitive or redundant to you. However, I need all of the answers to come directly from you, even if I may already know the answer. We must be consistent with each patient to minimize any possibility of bias. Also, remember that there are **no wrong answers.***

TINNITUS

*The first series of questions are specific to your **tinnitus**. Please think only about your **tinnitus** when you answer these questions.*

1. Do you have "bad days" when your tinnitus is particularly bothersome, or does it seem equally bothersome from day to day?

☐ No, doesn't have "bad days"—**Go to Question 2**

☐ Yes, has "bad days"—How often do you have these "bad days?"

☐ 1	*days per*	☐ Week
☐ 2		☐ Month
☐ 3		☐ Year
☐ 4		
☐ 5 or more		

(If YES) Do you have these bad days "more often," "less often," or "just as often" as you did before you started treatment?

☐ More often ☐ Less often ☐ Just as often ☐ Not sure

(If YES) Are your bad days "the same," "not as bad," or "worse" than before you started treatment?

☐ The same ☐ Not as bad ☐ Worse ☐ Not sure

2. Do sounds ever cause a change in the loudness of your tinnitus?

☐ No effect—**Go to Question 3**
☐ Softer—**Go to Question 3**
☐ Louder

(If LOUDER) What kinds of sounds cause this change? **(Interviewer:** Ask as an open-ended question; do not read list to patient; check all categories that apply)

☐ **Very loud sounds/activities** that would be expected to cause a change in the loudness of tinnitus (e.g., firing a gun, attending a concert, using power tools)
☐ **Higher pitched sounds** (e.g., squeals, squeaks, beeps, whistles, rings)
☐ **Lower pitched sounds** (e.g., bass from radio)
☐ **Traffic (warning) sounds** (e.g., emergency vehicle sirens, car horns, back-up beeper on truck/van)
☐ **Traffic (background) sounds** (e.g., road noise, road construction, diesel engines, garbage trucks)
☐ **Sudden impact sounds** (e.g., door slam, car backfiring, objects dropping on floor, dishes clattering)
☐ **Voices** (e.g., television, radio, movies, children's voices, dog barking)
☐ **Other** (describe) ______________________________

When any of these sounds cause your tinnitus to change, how long does the change last?

☐ 1–2	☐ Seconds
☐ 3–4	☐ Minutes
☐ 5–10	☐ Hours
☐ more than 10	☐ Days

When you hear a sound that causes your tinnitus to change, does the effect sometimes last until the next morning after you've slept?

☐ No—**Go to Question 3**
☐ Yes

(If EFFECT LASTS AT LEAST UNTIL THE NEXT MORNING) What kinds of sounds cause this to happen? **(Interviewer:** Ask as an open-ended question; do not read list to patient; check all categories that apply)

☐ **Very loud sounds/activities** (e.g., firing a gun, attending a concert, using power tools)
☐ **Higher pitched sounds** (e.g., squeals, squeaks, beeps, whistles, rings)
☐ **Lower pitched sounds** (e.g., bass from radio)
☐ **Traffic (warning) sounds** (e.g., emergency vehicle sirens, car horns, back-up beeper on truck/van)
☐ **Traffic (background) sounds** (e.g., road noise, road construction, diesel engines, garbage trucks)
☐ **Sudden impact sounds** (e.g., door slam, car backfiring, objects dropping on floor, dishes clattering)
☐ **Voices** (e.g., television, radio, movies, children's voices, dog barking)
☐ **Other** (describe) ______________________________

3. Do you use ear protection (earplugs or earmuffs)?

☐ No—**Go to Question 4**
☐ Yes

(If YES) Why do you use ear protection?

☐ To keep tinnitus from getting louder
☐ Trouble tolerating everyday sounds that seem normal to others
☐ Other ______________________________

(**Interviewer:** Determine if the patient uses ear protection specifically because of tinnitus—this would usually be to prevent the tinnitus from getting louder, which should not be suggested to the patient to avoid "negative counseling." Also, determine if the patient uses ear protection specifically because of trouble tolerating environmental sounds that seem normal to others—this too should not be suggested to avoid negative counseling. Other reasons for using ear protection do not need to be recorded.)

IF EAR PROTECTION IS USED FOR TINNITUS: What percent of the time do you use earplugs or earmuffs **for your tinnitus**?

☐ 5%	☐ 30%	☐ 55%	☐ 80%
☐ 10%	☐ 35%	☐ 60%	☐ 85%
☐ 15%	☐ 40%	☐ 65%	☐ 90%
☐ 20%	☐ 45%	☐ 70%	☐ 95%
☐ 25%	☐ 50%	☐ 75%	☐ 100%

Do you use your earplugs or earmuffs **for your tinnitus** when it's fairly quiet?
☐ No
☐ Yes

Interviewer: Does patient **overprotect** ears because of tinnitus? (if so, discuss importance of not overprotecting)
☐ No
☐ Yes

4. Are you currently receiving any other treatment specifically for your tinnitus?
☐ No—**Go to Question 5**
☐ Yes

(If YES) What?

☐ Herbs	☐ Counseling
☐ Vitamins	☐ Tabletop sound machines
☐ Hypnosis	☐ Special CDs or tapes
☐ Acupuncture	☐ Other ________________

5. What is the **biggest reason** your tinnitus is a problem (not including trouble hearing or trouble understanding speech)

____

6. I'm going to read through a list of activities and I want you to tell me how often your tinnitus keeps you from doing these activities, or how often it negatively affects these activities in any way. Please don't include trouble hearing or trouble understanding speech when you answer these questions.

	Never	**Rarely**	**Sometimes**	**Often**	**Always**	**N/A**
a. Concentration?	☐	☐	☐	☐	☐	☐
b. Sleep?	☐	☐	☐	☐	☐	☐
c. Quiet resting activities (reading, relaxing, etc.)?	☐	☐	☐	☐	☐	☐

(**Interviewer:** For questions d through i, if the patient reports an effect from tinnitus, ask the patient **how** or **why** the activity is affected. You do not need to record how or why the activity is affected—this is asked to ensure that the patient is not including hearing difficulties in the responses.)

	Never	Rarely	Sometimes	Often	Always	N/A
d. Work? (select N/A if retired)	☐	☐	☐	☐	☐	☐
e. Day-to-day responsibilities outside of work?	☐	☐	☐	☐	☐	☐
f. Going to restaurants?	☐	☐	☐	☐	☐	☐
g. Participating in or observing sports events?	☐	☐	☐	☐	☐	☐
h. Social activities?	☐	☐	☐	☐	☐	☐
i. Anything else? ________________	☐	☐	☐	☐	☐	☐

7. What percent of your **total awake time**, over the last month, were you **noticing or thinking about** your tinnitus? Please give an average percentage over the last month.

☐ 5%	☐ 30%	☐ 55%	☐ 80%
☐ 10%	☐ 35%	☐ 60%	☐ 85%
☐ 15%	☐ 40%	☐ 65%	☐ 90%
☐ 20%	☐ 45%	☐ 70%	☐ 95%
☐ 25%	☐ 50%	☐ 75%	☐ 100%

Has this percentage changed since the beginning of treatment?
☐ No
☐ Yes—How much do you think it has changed? ________%

(**Interviewer**: Indicate patient's response from the Initial Interview ________%)

8. What percent of your **total awake time**, over the last month, were you **annoyed, distressed, or irritated** by your tinnitus? Please give an average percentage over the last month.

☐ 5%	☐ 30%	☐ 55%	☐ 80%
☐ 10%	☐ 35%	☐ 60%	☐ 85%
☐ 15%	☐ 40%	☐ 65%	☐ 90%
☐ 20%	☐ 45%	☐ 70%	☐ 95%
☐ 25%	☐ 50%	☐ 75%	☐ 100%

Has this percentage changed since the beginning of treatment?
☐ No
☐ Yes—How much do you think it has changed? ________%

(**Interviewer**: Indicate patient's response from the Initial Interview ________%)

(**Interviewer**: Double-check that patient responded appropriately to Questions 7 and 8, i.e., to *total awake time for each condition of* ***awareness*** *and* ***annoyance****, respectively*)

I'm now going to ask you to rank your tinnitus, on a scale of 0 to 10, with regard to severity, annoyance, and effect on your life. Please do not include trouble hearing or trouble understanding speech when you answer these questions.

*(**Interviewer**: Underline patient's previous responses for questions 9, 10, and 11; telling patients "improvement" is okay, but don't tell them previous numbers)*

9. How **strong**, or **loud**, was your tinnitus, on average, over the last month? "0" would be "no tinnitus"; "10" would be "as loud as you can imagine."

(no tinnitus)	**0**	**1**	**2**	**3**	**4**	**5**	**6**	**7**	**8**	**9**	**10**	**(as loud as imaginable)**

10. How much has tinnitus **annoyed you**, on average, over the last month—not including annoyance from trouble hearing or trouble understanding speech? "0" would be "not annoying at all"; "10" would be "as annoying as you can imagine."

(not annoying)	**0**	**1**	**2**	**3**	**4**	**5**	**6**	**7**	**8**	**9**	**10**	**(as annoying as imaginable)**

11. How much did tinnitus **affect or impact your life**, on average, over the last month—not including impact from trouble hearing or trouble understanding speech? "0" would be "not at all"; "10" would be "as much as you can imagine."

(no impact)	**0**	**1**	**2**	**3**	**4**	**5**	**6**	**7**	**8**	**9**	**10**	**(as much impact as imaginable)**

12. Do you have any other comments about your tinnitus? ______________________

SOUND TOLERANCE

(**Interviewer**: Ask these questions only if patient had a sound tolerance problem at the initial visit)

*The next series of questions is only about your **ability to tolerate sound**. Please think only about **sound tolerance** when you answer these questions.*

13. Describe the sounds that cause you pain or physical discomfort. (**Interviewer**: Ask as an open-ended question; do not read list to patient; check all categories that apply)

- ☐ **Higher pitched sounds** (e.g., squeals, squeaks, beeps, whistles, rings)
- ☐ **Lower pitched sounds** (e.g., bass from radio)
- ☐ **Traffic (warning) sounds** (e.g., emergency vehicle sirens, car horns, back-up beeper on truck/van)
- ☐ **Traffic (background) sounds** (e.g., road noise, road construction, diesel engines, garbage trucks)
- ☐ **Sudden impact sounds** (e.g., door slam, car backfiring, objects dropping on floor, dishes clattering)
- ☐ **Voices** (e.g., television, radio, movies, children's voices, dog barking)
- ☐ **Other** (describe) ______________________

14. Do you have "bad days" when sound tolerance is more of a problem than on other days, or is your ability to tolerate sound the same from day to day?

- ☐ No, doesn't have "bad days"—**Go to Question 15**
- ☐ Yes, has "bad days"—How often do you have these "bad days?"

☐ 1	*days per*	☐ Week
☐ 2		☐ Month
☐ 3		☐ Year
☐ 4		
☐ 5 or more		

(If YES) Do you have these bad days "more often," "less often," or "just as often" as before you started treatment?

☐ More often ☐ Less often ☐ Just as often ☐ Not sure

(If YES) Are your bad days "the same," "not as bad," or "worse" than before you started treatment?

☐ The same ☐ Not as bad ☐ Worse ☐ Not sure

15. Do sounds ever cause a change in how much sound you can tolerate?

☐ No effect—**Go to Question 16**
☐ Better able to tolerate sound—**Go to Question 16**
☐ Less able to tolerate sound

(If LESS ABLE TO TOLERATE SOUND) What kinds of sounds have this effect? **(Interviewer:** Ask as an open-ended question; do not read list to patient; check all categories that apply)

☐ **Very loud sounds/activities** (e.g., firing a gun, attending a concert, using power tools
☐ **Higher pitched sounds** (e.g., squeals, squeaks, beeps, whistles, rings)
☐ **Lower pitched sounds** (e.g., bass from radio)
☐ **Traffic (warning) sounds** (e.g., emergency vehicle sirens, car horns, back-up beeper on truck/van)
☐ **Traffic (background) sounds** (e.g., road noise, road construction, diesel engines, garbage trucks)
☐ **Sudden impact sounds** (e.g., door slam, car backfiring, objects dropping on floor, dishes clattering)
☐ **Voices** (e.g., television, radio, movies, children's voices, dog barking)
☐ **Other** (describe) ______________________________

When any of these sounds reduce your sound tolerance, how long does the change last?

☐ 1–2 ☐ Seconds
☐ 3–4 ☐ Minutes
☐ 5–10 ☐ Hours
☐ more than 10 ☐ Days

When you hear a sound that reduces your ability to tolerate sounds, does the effect sometimes last until the next morning after you've slept?

☐ No—**Go to Question 16**
☐ Yes

(IF EFFECT LASTS AT LEAST UNTIL NEXT MORNING) What kinds of sounds cause this to happen? **(Interviewer:** Ask as an open-ended question; do not read list to patient; check all categories that apply)

☐ **Very loud sounds/activities** (e.g., firing a gun, attending a concert, using power tools)
☐ **Higher pitched sounds** (e.g., squeals, squeaks, beeps, whistles, rings)
☐ **Lower pitched sounds** (e.g., bass from radio)
☐ **Traffic (warning) sounds** (e.g., emergency vehicle sirens, car horns, back-up beeper on truck/van)
☐ **Traffic (background) sounds** (e.g., road noise, road construction, diesel engines, garbage trucks)
☐ **Sudden impact sounds** (e.g., door slam, car backfiring, objects dropping on floor, dishes clattering)
☐ **Voices** (e.g., television, radio, movies, children's voices, dog barking)
☐ **Other** (describe) ______________________________

16. (**Interviewer:** In Question 3 did the patient report the use of hearing protection because of "trouble tolerating everyday sounds"?)

☐ No—**Go to Question 17**
☐ Yes

(If YES) Earlier you told me that you sometimes use ear protection because of trouble tolerating sound—what percent of the time do you use ear protection **because of that trouble**?

☐ 5% ☐ 30% ☐ 55% ☐ 80%
☐ 10% ☐ 35% ☐ 60% ☐ 85%
☐ 15% ☐ 40% ☐ 65% ☐ 90%
☐ 20% ☐ 45% ☐ 70% ☐ 95%
☐ 25% ☐ 50% ☐ 75% ☐ 100%

(If YES) Do you use your earplugs when it's fairly quiet **because of trouble tolerating sound**?

☐ No
☐ Yes

(**Interviewer**: Does patient **overprotect** ears **due to problems with sound tolerance**?)

☐ No
☐ Yes

17. Are you currently receiving any treatment specifically for problems with **sound tolerance**?

☐ No—**Go to Question 18**
☐ Yes

(If YES) What?

☐ Herbs ☐ Counseling
☐ Vitamins ☐ Tabletop sound machines
☐ Hypnosis ☐ Special CDs or tapes
☐ Acupuncture ☐ Other ________________

18. I'm going to read a list of activities and I want you to tell me how often trouble tolerating sound keeps you from doing these activities, or how often it negatively affects these activities in any way.

(**Interviewer:** Underline patient's previous responses. Telling patients "improvement" is okay, but don't tell them previous answers. Check only one box for each activity.)

	Never	Rarely	Sometimes	Often	Always	N/A
a. Concerts?	☐	☐	☐	☐	☐	☐
b. Shopping?	☐	☐	☐	☐	☐	☐
c. Movies?	☐	☐	☐	☐	☐	☐
d. Work? (select N/A if retired)	☐	☐	☐	☐	☐	☐
e. Day-to-day responsibilities outside of work?	☐	☐	☐	☐	☐	☐
f. Going to restaurants?	☐	☐	☐	☐	☐	☐
g. Driving?	☐	☐	☐	☐	☐	☐
h. Participating in or observing sports events?	☐	☐	☐	☐	☐	☐
i. Attending church?	☐	☐	☐	☐	☐	☐
j. Housekeeping activities?	☐	☐	☐	☐	☐	☐
k. Child care?	☐	☐	☐	☐	☐	☐
l. Social activities?	☐	☐	☐	☐	☐	☐
m. Anything else? ________________	☐	☐	☐	☐	☐	☐

I'm now going to ask you to rank your ***sound tolerance****, on a scale of 0 to 10, with regard to severity, annoyance, and effect on your life.*

(**Interviewer**: Underline patient's previous responses for questions 19, 20, and 21. Telling patients "improvement" is okay, but don't tell them the previous numbers.)

19. First, I'd like you to rate your ability to tolerate sound on a scale of "0" to "10." "0" would mean "you can tolerate all sounds"; "10" would mean "you cannot tolerate any sounds."

(can tolerate all) **0 1 2 3 4 5 6 7 8 9 10** **(cannot tolerate any)**

20. How much has trouble tolerating sound **annoyed you**, on average, over the last month? "0" would be "not annoying at all"; "10" would be "as annoying as you can imagine."

(not annoying) **0 1 2 3 4 5 6 7 8 9 10** **(as annoying as imaginable)**

21. How much did trouble tolerating sound affect your life, on average, over the last month? "0" would be "not at all"; "10" would be "as much as you can imagine."

(not at all) **0 1 2 3 4 5 6 7 8 9 10** **(as much as imaginable)**

22. Do you have any other comments about trouble tolerating sound?

____

HEARING

23. Do you think you have a hearing problem?

☐ No
☐ Yes
☐ Not sure

RANKING PROBLEMS

(**Interviewer**: Underline patient's previous responses for questions 24, 25, and 26. Telling patients "improvement" is okay, but don't tell them the previous numbers.)

24. How much of a problem is **tinnitus** (if you are not including problems from trouble hearing or trouble understanding speech)? "0" would be "no problem at all"; "10" would be "as much as you can imagine."

(no problem) **0 1 2 3 4 5 6 7 8 9 10** **(as much as imaginable)**

25. How much of a problem is **trouble tolerating sound**? "0" would be "no problem at all"; "10" would be "as much as you can imagine."

(no problem) **0 1 2 3 4 5 6 7 8 9 10** **(as much as imaginable)**

26. How much of a problem is **hearing**? "0" would be "no problem at all"; "10" would be "as much as you can imagine."

(no problem)	**0**	**1**	**2**	**3**	**4**	**5**	**6**	**7**	**8**	**9**	**10**	**(as much as imaginable)**

27. Next I'd like you to tell me if you are doing the same, better, or worse with each of the issues we have talked about.

(**Interviewer:** Do not ask the patient about trouble tolerating sound or about hearing if these were not identified as problems.)

	Same	**Better**	**Worse**	**N/A**
a. Tinnitus	☐	☐	☐	☐
b. Trouble tolerating sound	☐	☐	☐	☐
c. Hearing	☐	☐	☐	☐

If you combine those issues, would you say your problem in general is the same, better, or worse than before you started treatment?

(**Interviewer:** Only ask this question if the patient has a problem with more than one of these issues.)

d. Problem in general	☐	☐	☐	☐

SUPPLEMENTAL QUESTIONS

28. How would you feel if you had to give back your instruments?

[**Interviewer:** (1) Ask as an open-ended question—do not read the response choices to the patient; (2) mark the box that **best** describes the patient's response; (3) emphasize to the patient that regardless of how this question is answered, the ear-level instruments will not be taken away.]

☐ They don't seem to be helping, but I'd be unhappy/upset about giving them back because I'd like to keep trying
☐ They don't seem to help and returning them wouldn't bother me
☐ They seem to be helping and I'd be unhappy/upset if I had to return them
☐ They've been helpful, but I don't need them anymore

29. Are you glad you started this program?
☐ No ☐ Yes ☐ Not sure

Interviewer:

(A) Indicate the main problems discussed during this interview:

____

(B) Recommendation: ________________________________

(C) Patient decision: ________________________________

(D) Next visit: ________________________________

Portions of this form adapted from Henry, J. A., Jastreboff, M. M., Jastreboff, P. J., Schechter, M. A., & Fausti, S. A. (2003); Henry, J A., Zaugg, T. L., & Schechter, M. A., (2005); and Jastreboff, P. J. & Hazell, J. W. P. (2004). Adapted with permission from the authors.

APPENDIX C

Patient Take-Home Reminders

TRT: Keys to Achieving Success

- Understand tinnitus and its benign nature
  - "Reclassify" tinnitus to the category of a neutral stimulus
- *Avoid silence*
  - "Enrich" your sound environment 24/7
- Adjust and use sound generators according to the protocol
- Attend all follow-up appointments
- With proper treatment, habituation usually takes 1 to 2 years

Sound Generators: Points to Remember

- Adjust the sound carefully in a quiet room
  - Adjust to a level close to but below the "mixing point" (just below the level at which the tinnitus sound starts to change)
  - Make sure the sound is below the level that could cause any annoyance or discomfort
- "Set and forget"
  - *Do not readjust* while they are in your ears
- Wear every day and as much as possible
- Enrich your sound environment 24/7
- If broken, return *immediately* for repair

Index

A

R

S

T